T0095455

What Do the Doctors Say?

How Doctors Create a World through Their Words

Janet Farrell Leontiou, Ph.D.

iUniverse, Inc.
New York   Bloomington

What Do the Doctors Say?
How Doctors Create a World through Their Words

Copyright © 20010 by Janet Farrell Leontiou, Ph.D.

All rights reserved. No part of this book may be used or reproduced by any means, graphic, electronic, or mechanical, including photocopying, recording, taping or by any information storage retrieval system without the written permission of the publisher except in the case of brief quotations embodied in critical articles and reviews.

iUniverse books may be ordered through booksellers or by contacting:
iUniverse
1663 Liberty Drive
Bloomington, IN 47403
www.iuniverse.com
1-800-Authors (1-800-288-4677)

Because of the dynamic nature of the Internet, any Web addresses or links contained in this book may have changed since publication and may no longer be valid. The views expressed in this work are solely those of the author and do not necessarily reflect the views of the publisher, and the publisher hereby disclaims any responsibility for them.

ISBN: 978-1-4502-2582-3 (pbk)
ISBN: 978-1-4502-2581-6 (ebk)
ISBN: 978-1-4502-2580-9 (hbk)

Library of Congress Control Number: 2010904979

Printed in the United States of America
iUniverse rev. date: 7/12/10

To Chris, Andreas, and Zachary,
who embody the meaning of agape

Contents

Acknowledgments

There are many people in my life who are very important and who have become a circle of supporters.

First, I want to thank our nanny, Alma, who makes all things possible.

Second, I wish to thank our son's therapists, who tirelessly work to teach him and encourage him. Every day, they do extraordinary work with grace and humor. The list is extensive: Laurie Dubner, Joe Kiefer, Terri Sperber, RoAnne Zuckerman, Jen Iasillo, Wendy Lager, Marcie Klebanoff, Anthony Quijano, Billy Ayres, Ailene Tisser, Mary Ellen Monteirro, Andrea Eckerley, and Kati Totne Racz. I owe them a huge debt of gratitude. Thank you also to Phil Schneider for being there.

Third, I want to express my gratitude to our school district. I am deeply grateful to Diane Santangelo and her staff for seeing Andreas as an individual and not just one more child with disabilities.

Fourth, I want to thank all the alternative health care professionals who helped us when traditional medicine could not.

Fifth, I wish to thank Jan Maslow for her very insightful comments about early parts of this work.

Sixth, thanks to Lisa Trump for her support—both tangible and intangible.

I have used the real names of the doctors who are exceptional: Dr. Ellen Manos, Dr. Amy Eisenberg, Dr. Cecelia McCarton, and Dr. John Pappas. For their care of our son, Andreas, thank you also to Dr. Stacey Zarakiotis and Dr. Sophie Poselle. I am very grateful for the professional services of Kathy Mitas and Edmund Simon at the Blood Lab at Greenwich Hospital.

Introduction

Before beginning my story, I want to introduce my sons, Andreas and Zachary. Zachary is a typically developing seven-year-old, and his twin brother, Andreas, carries a diagnosis of cerebral palsy. I say that Andreas carries the diagnosis because I am not convinced that Andreas has cerebral palsy. He has multiple disabilities, and I have no other label that seems to fit. Finding the correct diagnosis is part of this journey, and I am not yet at its end. When naming the boys, my husband and I chose the alpha and the omega to designate our first and last sons and to reflect their Greek heritage. Now, their names reflect the span between them and their different experiences. Raising a typically developing child, like Zachary, is pretty straightforward. Raising a child like Andreas, however, presents multiple challenges. This book mentions some of the difficulties we regularly face, but these day-to-day challenges are not the main focus. This book addresses the difficulties that come from the necessary interactions with the medical community.

I am a professor of communication, and since I had my son, I have noticed that the medical culture has its own language when it comes to disability. I call this the "discourse of disability." This discourse does not involve blatant violations of political correctness; the goal of this book goes beyond such notions. I am not speaking about doctors using the label "cripple" to refer to my son. Everyone knows that this label is no longer appropriate.

I am instead speaking about something deeper that involves all of us. I want to provide a step-by-step description of how we all participate in creating a mythology concerning doctors and medicine.

We produce mythologies through our talk. The word *myth* is Greek, and it means "a telling." It does not mean something false but instead refers to how we talk about something. The way we talk about someone or something determines how both we and our listeners experience that person or thing. For instance, most corporations have foundation myths that tell about how the company began. Sometimes people from outside the company even know the foundation myths; for example, we've all heard that clothing designer Ralph Lauren began by selling neckties or that the computer companies Apple and Microsoft began in garages. Neither truth nor falsehood pertains to these stories; rather, these are the ways we speak about the beginnings of these companies. In this book, how we speak about something is what I mean by myth.

Hopefully, parents who are raising children with disabilities will recognize my story because it is not mine alone. I want parents to know that if they have a sense that something is wrong in the way that doctors speak to them, those feelings are legitimate. The medical culture, like most cultures, makes sense to those who live within it. I hope to tell my story in a context that resonates for others and provides parents with language to talk about their experiences.

A person who has the language to speak about her or his experience has the power to change the nature of the dialogue. While the discourse of disability is pervasive and has significant ramifications that spiral out and affect the therapeutic as well as the educational community, once parents understand how the discourse works, they can change their own participation in it and advocate for change.

The Rhetoric of Connection

Over the last twenty to thirty years, developed countries have undergone tremendous positive changes in their treatment of children with disabilities. Many U.S. states' departments of health and human resources have created a program called Early Intervention in response to parents of children with disabilities who contended that the current medical model was failing to serve their children. A therapy-based model, EI is an incredible opportunity for children, zero to three years of age, to receive therapies within their home.

I am proposing another shift. Many of the difficulties that I encounter as a parent of a child with disabilities would be lessened if I encountered more health care professionals who practiced connection—connection to themselves as people, connection to the child, connection to the parent, and connection to the other modalities of treatment that are available. I call this shift "the rhetoric of connection."

The way a person speaks creates either connection or disconnection. Words have the power to create our own reality— both for the speaker and the listener. In my academic work, I have tried to make sense of my own experience. I try to use what I have been taught about language to create a cohesive narrative about medical culture and its impact on the health care consumer. This narrative may apply to all of us but I am especially interested in those aspects that apply to children with disabilities.

We create worlds through our words and then act as if those worlds are not our creation. How we speak about something makes it appear natural and God-given instead of manufactured through our talk. One function that myth provides is to remove the onus of responsibility. If no one has created a situation, no one need take responsibility. In part, we accomplish this lack of responsibility through grammatical structure. Instead of saying, "I made a mistake," the doctor, looking to avoid blame, may state, "Mistakes have happened."

One phrase decidedly indicates myth making: "That's the way it is." This phrase suggests that the current practice (whatever it may be) has always been and will always remain. The speaker insinuates that the situation at hand was not created by anyone and, therefore, cannot be changed.

Disconnection in the Medical Community

The following is a list of characteristics of medical culture, not exhaustive, but rather an illustration of how talk creates a culture:

The doctor is the only one who knows.

o Parents of the patient may be perceived as obstacles. The medical community is a locked-in and self-contained system. Medical culture induces inhabitants to maintain the status quo. Cultural members are, at times, oblivious to the effect that their words have on others outside of the culture. The culture is impervious to criticism from those outside the medical culture.

o   Some of the patient's symptoms may be explained away by a reference to the primary diagnosis. Medical practitioners often exaggerate their own importance.

I am aware that this list is not complimentary. I am, however, revealing how we all participate in maintaining this mythology of the medical community, even though it does not serve us as patients. One reason why we recreate this mythology is the pull, on all of us, to maintain the status quo. We sometimes work to keep things the same, even if they're harmful. For instance, parents may recreate their parents' familiar parenting practices rather than choose parenting practices based on what they feel is best. Change can be threatening. All of us—health care professionals and patients—suffer in the existing system. Yet, all of us are drawn into ensuring the culture's survival.

This book's title comes from a question I've heard again and again since Andreas was born: What do the doctors say? How to answer is always a challenge for me. Perhaps, here, I can start by pointing out that the simple asking of the question maintains the myth that doctors are the only ones who know. I also hope to provide an analysis of what doctors literally say.

If I had to use one word to describe the medical culture, it would be *disconnected*.

In seeking care for our son, I have encountered too many doctors who seem disconnected from their patients, their patients' parents, their colleagues, and other areas of treatment. For each chapter, I have outlined the type of disconnection that is occurring through the doctors' talk. Disconnection can occur when the doctor is so preoccupied by a computer screen that he or she barely looks at the patient. Disconnection can occur between the doctor and the parent when the doctor uses dismissive language toward the parent. Disconnection can occur when a hospital assigns an intern—sans introduction to or permission from a patient or the patient's family—to shadow a physician as he or she treats patients. This disconnect occurs when a doctor allows anyone in an examination room without first asking the patient's permission. At the very least, the doctor should introduce the intern to the patient and explain the purpose of his or her presence. Another form of disconnect occurs when a doctor appears completely unaware of all complementary modalities of treatment. I do not think that doctors must be completely informed about treatments that fall outside of traditional medicine. I do think that patients and parents would appreciate doctors who demonstrate knowledge that alternatives exist, avoid speaking disparagingly about that which they do not know, and acknowledge their own lack of knowledge.

In this book, I will provide parents with a language to speak about the culture of disconnection they may encounter. The language is necessary because you cannot speak about—or, arguably, even think about—something without a vocabulary in which to do so. For the sake of analogy, let's use the term sexual harassment. In our grandparent's time, there was no language for speaking about this practice. If an individual did experience sexual harassment, he or she probably would have described what occurred (if at all) as "that's just the way it is." Now we have a language to speak about this practice, and we have laws enacted to try to prevent it.

I have created a list of language patterns germane to the medical culture I am describing. I have given each of these patterns a label so that, if you are in a similar circumstance, you'll be able to label your experience and speak about the experience to others. These language patterns include the language of self-importance, the destructive metaphor, the use and abuse of labels, the language of unilateral action, language that constructs the caregiver as an obstacle, the language of contradiction, the language of ambiguity, thoughtless language, the language of the self-contained system, the language of condescension, the language of generalization, and the language of passive aggression.

As I've encountered the medical culture, I've found it to be highly subjective, even though medicine holds itself up as an objective enterprise. Within the disability literature, written mostly by mothers, a common refrain is the frustration of encountering doctors who masquerade opinions behind the veil of objective fact. Martha Beck, in *Expecting Adam*, speaks about the experience in this way: "Oh, I'm sorry—do I sound bitter? Hm. Perhaps that's because … I have had so many physicians wedge their personal prejudices into my life, into Adam's life, and call it medical advice" (Beck 2000).

Chapter 1
The Language of Self-importance
or "The *I*'s Have It"

Disconnected from the Parent in the Therapeutic Setting

Early on in my entrance into the medical/therapeutic world, I encountered the "language of self-importance." One of the first lessons I received on the language of self-importance involved Andreas's walker. Andreas started using a walker when he was about three years old. I researched several types of walkers, printed out specs sheet on each brand, helped to identify which one would work best for Andreas, got the prescription for the walker from his pediatrician, and attained a loaner so that Andreas could try one out. I then brought everything that I had to his physical therapist, Tina.

I remember sitting at a school meeting for Andreas when Tina said, "I secured a walker for Andreas." Everyone, including my husband, congratulated her on her accomplishment. I was in an uncomfortable position. I had done much of the work for getting my son the walker, but if I pointed that out, I would sound petty. I was happy to do the work, but I realized during that meeting how the system was set up to exclude me. I made a comment to my husband about how things had gone behind the scenes. My hunch was then and still is that, in most cases involving disabled children, the mother drives the process for the child's treatment and care, but when it comes to acknowledgment, she is invisible. My husband's response was bottom-line driven: "You got the desired outcome. I don't understand why you're complaining."

I am interested in how talk creates the impression that a single person, the professional, is driving the process rather than it being a cooperative effort. I am also interested in how the mother's efforts usually get shut out. I have found that the mothers I know usually go along with this charade because, in the end, they most care about services for their child and not who gets the credit. The professionals give the impression that they are working unilaterally, and that ensures their own sense of professional worth.

What I find most striking is that, when I reflect on the good interventions that I have brought to my son, most have been recommendations from other mothers. Doctors don't offer many ideas for navigating the world of disability. Yet, I am repeatedly asked, "What do the doctors say?" I don't know exactly how to answer this question. Rather, I'm interested in examining how asking the question places the doctor in a central position and gives the impression that the doctor is the only one who knows. I have never been asked, "What do other parents who are in your circumstance say?"

Most parents who have a child with a disability will identify with my frustration surrounding the fact that every intervention must begin with a doctor's prescription. Most pediatricians are outside the day-to-day care of a child with disability, yet insurance companies insist that all requests, for anything from therapy to equipment, start with a prescription from the doctor.

We all play a role in establishing the doctor as authority through our talk. Once when Andreas had a seizure after being seizure-free for five years, I kept him home and canceled his therapy schedule. A friend asked, "Did the doctor tell you to do that?" Again, I was faced with a dilemma as to how to respond. If I spoke the truth, I would sound arrogant. I was the one making the decisions as to what Andreas most needed. The question, again, created the impression that a doctor behind the scene was directing a plan of treatment and I was following along. Most doctors are too busy and see too many patients to be that involved in the care of their patients, yet the mythology remains.

We all may play a role in recreating this mythology because we want the security that someone, other than ourselves, is really in charge. Speaking with a friend about a potential new neurologist, I mentioned that the doctor provided us with a new diagnosis. She said, "It sounds like you found a good captain."

I responded, "It sounds like I may have found a good first mate."

I think my friend may have interpreted my response as hostile. I am not looking for anyone to be the captain, but I could use some help running the ship. I know that, ultimately, I take responsibility for the course we are on.

When Andreas had the seizure, I called his pediatrician's office, and the receptionist told me to come in. We met with an unfamiliar pediatrician in the practice because Andreas's primary doctor was not in. She asked me to describe what happened. When I had finished, she told me, "I think you are right. I think that he had a seizure. I think that you need to go see a neurologist."

I knew what I had witnessed because Andreas seized during the first weeks after birth, and for many days, I held him in the NICU (Neonatal Intensive Care Unit) as he seized repeatedly. We went to see Dr. Phillips.

Dr. Phillips turned out to be different from most doctors we had visited. We went directly from the pediatrician's office to Dr. Phillips' office. After I explained what had happened, Dr. Phillips asked me a question I have never before been asked by a physician: "What do you think happened?"

I explained that I thought Andreas's brain had reset itself.

He then asked, "Do you say that out of intuition or knowledge?"

I answered that my response was a little bit of both. I had read about the brain resetting itself, and I felt that this is what happened with Andreas.

Dr. Philips went on to talk about how the phenomenon of the brain resetting itself was documented in the literature. Dr. Phillips also did not think that Andreas had cerebral palsy because he did not experience the preconditions that usually go along with the diagnosis. He looked at Andreas's smiling face and suggested that he may have Angelman syndrome. AS is a genetic disorder, and smiling is one of the characteristics of the disorder. Subsequently, I had Andreas genetically tested for Angelman and the results were negative.

I told Andreas's therapists about the possibility of the diagnosis of AS, and they immediately dismissed it. Children with Angelman syndrome do smile a lot, which Andreas does, but their smiles are frozen and not in response to situations. Andreas's smiles, the therapists commented, are appropriate reactions to situations. His smile is not frozen.

I do not fault Dr. Phillips for getting it wrong. He was basing his diagnosis on one visit, and at least he was entertaining other possibilities besides the catch-all *cerebral palsy*. Thankfully, Andreas has not had another seizure since then, and I continue to see Dr. Phillips as someone I trust. I trust him because he is one of a handful of doctors who listens to me.

Disconnected from the Parent in the Hospital Setting

My experience with Dr. Phillips stands out because it was the only time that a physician asked my opinion. Unfortunately, not all of our experiences with neurologists were as positive. At the NICU, we crossed paths with Dr. Wellby. I had just given birth to twins via a caesarean section. I would leave one son at home with our nanny, and I would commute to Manhattan every day to be with Andreas. I would arrive in the morning, take my station in the rocking chair by his isolette, and rock him. One day, the nurse told me that Dr. Wellby was on the phone and wanted to talk to me. Dr. Wellby informed me that he wanted to perform a second spinal tap on Andreas. I told him that I did not know if I would approve a second spinal tap, since they already performed one and found nothing. I asked him why he didn't do a more comprehensive test during the first procedure. Dr. Wellby responded, "I am the doctor, and I will do what I think is necessary. There are other hospitals with which I am affiliated where I do not need parental consent to perform tests on babies.

I cannot test for everything under the sun with one test." So much for bedside manner.

Dr. Wellby did the second spinal tap and found nothing.

I know that I'm on shaky ground here. Doctors need to do procedures that the layperson may not understand or the parent may question the efficacy of. I do think that the doctor had a responsibility to teach me in that moment. This was an extremely difficult time for me, and Dr. Wellby, because of how he chose to speak to me, made it worse.

Dr. Wellby also told me that pain for a newborn is not the same as pain for an adult. He was suggesting that babies do not feel pain as acutely as adults. My common sense tells me that newborns experience pain more acutely because their nervous systems are immature. This point of view is articulated by Dr. Ricardo Carbajal, professor of pediatrics and chief of the National Center of Resources to Fight Pain at Children's Hospital Armand Trousseau in Paris, France. Dr. Carbajal states that neonates (babies from one to four weeks old) are more sensitive to pain, and prolonged exposure to pain may alter the way their brains function (Gordon 2008).

We visited Dr. Wellby one more time after Andreas was released from the hospital. I was instructed to follow up with him after release. During the visit, he exhibited the same bedside manner as he had in the hospital, and his office was filthy. We never saw him again.

Andreas was placed on anticonvulsive medications for the first year of his life. We saw another neurologist, Dr. Grains, during this time so that his medications could be monitored.

Seeing this doctor was benign—not particularly helpful but not caustic like our experience with Dr. Wellby.

After Andreas had remained seizure free and we had not seen Dr. Grains for some time, his pediatrician suggested that he see a neurologist regularly. We had not sought out another neurologist after Andreas came off the anticonvulsants because I did not see the purpose. Our pediatrician recommended that we see Dr. Spencer, so I scheduled an appointment. Dr. Spencer was congenial and listened well. I asked him directly what value he brought to us for Andreas's overall care. He told me that he could let us know of advances in research. This proved not to be the case. I called Dr. Spencer with questions about a research finding I had heard about and wondered if it could apply to Andreas. He said that he would look into it and call me back. He never did. The medical culture works in such a way that it does not acknowledge its own gaps in knowledge (like alternative methods to traditional health care) and sometimes there is no follow-up in the areas of expertise that physicians claim as their own (as in this case regarding the research). This experience with Dr. Grains is noteworthy because, while the medical culture maintains that the doctor is the only one who knows, the doctor is at times not very willing to share his or her expertise with a layperson.

After our visit, Dr. Spencer sent a report addressed to Andreas's pediatrician, which reiterated Andreas's story that I told him in his office. Every doctor who subsequently received that report expressed how thorough the report was. I provided the details of the report. Dr. Spencer was a good note taker. For this service, he charged six hundred dollars. Doctors frequently congratulate each other on their sole accomplishments without any hint of collaborative effort. In this case, I paid to have my own words validated. The doctor presented these words as if they were his own. In fact, my name is conspicuously absent from the report. The important point here is not that my ego suffered but that the medical culture only wants to accept as valid information or knowledge that comes from other professionals within the health care system.

Chapter 2
The Destructive Metaphor or "Evening out the Workload"

Disconnected from Awareness of One's Words in the Doctor's Office

In order to decipher any culture, it's important to pay close attention to the culture's language, particularly its use of metaphors. Metaphors aren't just figures of speech; they're figures of thought. Metaphors take our minds to a new place. The function of a metaphor is to shift our thinking. The origin of the word *metaphor* is Greek; it comes from *metaphorein*, meaning to move from one place to another place. Here I will talk about some the metaphors I encountered before the babies were conceived. The metaphors I will speak about come from a doctor working in the field of in vitro fertilization (IVF).

My husband and I tried to conceive for a long time. We were married for twenty-two years before the boys were born. When I was in my thirties, I discovered that I had a condition called endometriosis—residual menstrual blood that does not get eliminated and instead can attach to any organ within the body.

The first infertility doctor we consulted, Dr. Isak, suggested that pregnancy would be a way to stave off the endometrioma (the mass attached to an ovary) from growing back after surgery. I had come to Dr. Isak because the doctor I was seeing at the time suggested that I respond to the condition by having one of my ovaries removed. I told Dr. Isak of the doctor's recommendation. He considered her recommendation outdated but he framed it this way: "She would not have suggested removing the ovary. You must have misunderstood." He later discussed it with my doctor, and he simply said that he found her position unbelievable. I do not think that the experience caused Dr. Isak to reexamine his immediate reaction and interpretation. When he had heard a prognosis with which he disagreed, he immediately thought that the patient must have gotten it wrong. He reacted this way, I think, because he is working under the cultural assumption that the doctor is the only one who knows. When confronted with a doctor potentially getting it wrong, he attributes it to a lack of understanding on the part of the patient.

We went through two in vitro fertilization cycles with Dr. Isak with no luck. We took a break from the drugs and doctors. A friend of mine suggested that we consult with another in vitro fertilization doctor. I took her advice and made an appointment with Dr. Rosa.

When we visited Dr. Rosa's office for the first time, business was very good.

The waiting room was full of couples about our ages who were trying hard to give each other the courtesy of anonymity in a public place. The waiting room was spacious and attractive. The walls were covered by an artist whose paintings we also owned.

Eng Tay is a Malaysian artist whose subjects are frequently couples and families.

My treatment by Dr. Rosa did not match the warm tones of the Eng Tay paintings. We saw Dr. Rosa enter the office and, from behind, I noticed a rolled-up *New York Post* sticking out of the back pocket of his pants. It is a small detail, but I remember noticing it. The newspaper is a sensational rag, the type with ridiculous headlines that you glance at while waiting to check out at the supermarket.

The IVF protocol is not for the faint of heart—for either member of the couple. There are the daily injections either self-administered or given by the partner, the side effects of the infertility drugs, and frequent doctor visits for monitoring. All of the difficulties are manageable, as long as you have the right kind of doctor. I was not so lucky.

I was trying to time my treatments so that the egg transfer would take place when was I was off from school. When undergoing IVF treatment, it is usual to begin hormone injections and, when the time is right, the eggs are extracted and fertilized. The fertilized eggs are then placed back into the woman's body. I had begun the hormone injections under the care of Dr. Rosa. One day, I received a call from his nurse telling me that Dr. Rosa wanted me to stay with the injections of Luperan—a drug I'd been taking since a previous surgery for endometriosis—for longer than I expected. I knew from previous experience that Luperan places the body into a false state of menopause where no eggs are produced. Only this time, I knew that there was no medical reason for staying on the drug. My hunch was that the doctor was suggesting this because of his convenience and schedule.

I called Dr. Rosa and explained that I wanted the procedure to coincide with my break from my teaching schedule and I did not want to take additional drugs for nonmedical reasons.

Dr. Rosa explained his dilemma: "I have all of these planes ready to take off from LaGuardia airport and I need to place some into a holding pattern. I have to even out the workload."

I called this the use of the destructive metaphor—Dr. Rosa's language reflected that he saw his patients as inanimate objects that he needed to rearrange for his convenience. If I was the airplane, Dr. Rosa was the air traffic controller, more interested in preventing crashes than seeing to the safety of the individual passengers onboard.

I asked my ob-gyn, Dr. Ellen Manos, to intervene on my behalf. Ellen is a childhood friend, and I felt childish asking her for help. I knew, however, that if I appealed to Ellen, she would have more sway with Dr. Rosa than I could. At the time, I thought it was important to finish the cycle. Within a short time after I spoke with Ellen, Dr. Rosa's nurse called me back to tell me that the doctor was instructing me to stop the Luperan and begin hormone injections. As the nurse was talking to me on the telephone, Dr. Rosa entered the room. In the background, I heard him say, "Tell her that she owes me big time."

When I went in for the follow-up office visit, I was waiting on the examination table when Dr. Rosa entered the room. I wanted to address what had happened so I said, "I understand that I owe you big time."

Dr. Rosa replied, "I don't want to talk about it."

Here I would shift the overarching metaphor at play. Dr. Rosa sounded less like an overworked bureaucrat and more like a petulant five-year-old who had not gotten his way.

Dr. Rosa provided me with information about how he saw me through the use of his metaphors. I should never have contributed to his vision of me by staying in his treatment. I thought that he had something that I needed at the time, so I overlooked how he spoke to me. That was a mistake. I do not know what effect the stress of the situation had on the cycle not being successful—maybe it did and maybe it did not.

After the debacle with Dr. Rosa, his medical practice asked me to meet with a psychologist. The purpose of the meeting was to debrief patients about the IVF experience. I started to tell the psychologist that I had a negative experience with Dr. Rosa. The psychologist told me, "We are not here to speak badly about the doctors. Sometimes women are bitter because they do not get pregnant, and they end up blaming the doctor."

I realized that there was very little I could say to this woman. The more I tried to explain my impressions, the more she attributed them to my bitterness. In communication, this is called a double bind. I was asked about my experience and when I began to speak about it, I was told that this was not the kind of feedback they were looking for. This double bind allowed the psychologist to solicit only responses that complimented the doctors.

The experience with Dr. Rosa provided the training ground for paying close attention to the use of metaphor. If you are the parent of a child with disability, you already know that many people use different metaphors to refer to your child. We, as a population, have learned to clean up our language, and the

---

use of "cripple," "lame," and even "handicapped" is no longer commonplace. The next example comes from our school district, and I use it to show that, even when people try to sound more inclusive, their language may produce the opposite effect. I also use metaphor to discuss how medical, therapeutic, and educational language can bleed into one another.

Disconnected from Awareness of One's Words within the Educational Setting

Our school district has been extremely decent and open-minded regarding the inclusion of Andreas. Andreas has a school program that was tailored for him. After I became disenchanted with the special education school he was attending, I asked the school district to treat his private therapies as his school equivalent. The school district has accommodated us, and we enjoy a real partnership in the goal of educating Andreas. Andreas is now in his third year of this ad hoc schedule, and he is thriving.

Well-intentioned people think they are being helpful, but sometimes their words create division. During the first meeting with the school district when I proposed my idea for Andreas's program, the Committee on Special Education was very supportive. A member of the committee suggested that Andreas join the music class once a week so that Andreas would have some experience socializing with his peers in a school setting. All of us thought the idea was brilliant. During the meeting for the second year of Andreas's program, Andreas's special education therapist, Laurie, suggested that we expand Andreas's exposure to the classroom and have him join the special education class for two hours a week. The same member who suggested Andreas join the music class was resistant. This committee member had expressed resistance to Andreas joining the special education class before. To her credit, I think that this person is supportive of Andreas. I think that she was trying to ensure that everyone's needs were being met by having Andreas join the class. She stated that she thought that Andreas's presence would be disruptive to the class. I offered my own observations about the music class that I witnessed the prior year: "I saw plenty of disruptions and none of them came from Andreas." The chair of the Committee on Special Education did not see the reason for the resistance, and Andreas joined the special education class that fall.

Andreas and Zachary were turning six years old that fall. During the summer, I had worked on arranging for a puppet troupe to visit the kids' classrooms. Our county was licensed to perform a puppet show with Kids on the Block puppets. Kids on the Block puppets are child-size puppets depicting various disabilities. The skits teach children about the disabilities and offer a safe place to ask questions. There would be no cost to the school district, and the show coincided perfectly with the county's mission of teaching inclusion.

I had wanted the puppets to visit the school prior to the kids' birthday because I wanted them to learn about physical disability prior to encountering children using wheelchairs, walkers, and crutches. I also wanted to protect Zachary from the burden of explanation. I did not him to have to explain to his friends why his brother used a wheelchair. I thought that was too much for him to carry during his sixth birthday party.

One day prior to the birthday, Laurie, Andreas, and I were exiting school as I heard someone call my name. It was the person from the committee who had expressed reservations about Andreas attending the special education class.

"I know that you've been working on bringing the puppets to school, and I wanted to tell you that is not necessary," she said.

This reaction surprised me since I thought that the puppet show would serve all the kids.

She then continued, "I don't know if the teachers will have the time to have the puppets pushed in."

I know that teachers face severe time constraints, but I thought that the puppet show would fit in nicely with the school's mandate to teach about different groups.

The committee member's next sentence stopped me: "I already visited the class that Andreas will join, and I have prepared them. I let them know that we will have a special visitor."

After the brief conversation, I told Laurie that this was not the message I had hoped for. I did not wish to see the children as being prepared for a special visitor. The metaphor of "special visitor" sounds otherworldly. I commented to Laurie that the label made it sound like Andreas was from another planet.

The professional was well-intentioned, but I thought her approach was wrong, and I did not understand her reluctance. I chose to ignore the negativity and appeal directly to the principal. The principal immediately embraced the idea, and the puppets came to school the next week. The show was a success. The children were attentive and asked thoughtful questions. Andreas joined Zachary's class that day and their nanny, my husband, and I were all present. The puppeteer working the puppet depicting cerebral palsy was a man with cerebral palsy who himself, like the puppet, used a wheelchair.

During the birthday party, one boy in Zachary's class asked, "Why is Andreas in that chair?"

All I said in reply was, "You remember the puppet show, right?"

The boy responded, "Oh yeah."

I tell this story because referring to Andreas as a special visitor is also a metaphor.

While it is not offensive, it sets him apart from the other kids. I do not argue that Andreas is like every other kid. He has severe physical disabilities that immediately set him apart from the other kids but why do we need to establish that division before he arrives? I do not want children to be prepared for his arrival. I would like for him to show up and for his disability to be explained to the kids while he is present. I also thought the puppets would establish a positive connotation for the topic of disabilities, and the kids could allow themselves to ask the puppets questions without being afraid. This was what happened for all the children in the class, with the exception of one little girl who was afraid of puppets!

The school district is working to create a place where Andreas belongs as much as any other child. In the two examples that I offered in this chapter, the physician and the member of the school community represented obstacles. In the first example, I should have paid greater attention to the metaphor the physician used because to continue seeing him was to join him in his objectification of me. The school member is in a different category. I do not know her reason for presenting obstacles, and happily, they were surmountable, but my impulse is to think that her intention was good. She was trying to do what was best for all involved—the students in the special education class, the students in the regular classes, the special education class, the special education teacher, the regular classroom teacher, and Andreas.

Chapter 3
The Use and Abuse of Labels
or "The Blame Game"

Disconnected from How a Parent May See Events Differently

I teach my students that a choice of words is a choice of worlds. The label I choose for something or someone shapes the perception for the listener and the speaker.

When I was pregnant, I was vomiting for nine months. The label "morning sickness" did not adequately describe my experience. The label morning sickness makes it seem like it ends by noon. It does not sound like something that lasted all day for the entire gestation period.

My ob-gyn suggested that I take medication for the nausea, but I refused because I was afraid of what the medications would do to the babies. In fact, this stoic mentality did not serve me in the hospital. I did not take the pain medication after the caesarian section, and as the nurse explained, this was compromising my body's ability to heal. So, I took the medication and could then stand upright. Once I could stand, I could then walk. The healing process began. Or at least, I began to heal physically.

On the night of the boys' birth, I experienced every physical symptom I had during pregnancy in the most extreme and intense form. It was a hellish night, but in the morning, I was symptom free. It was as if my body was ridding itself of all the side effects from the pregnancy.

What I did not know that night was that my hellish experience was just beginning.

The boys were delivered via a caesarean section and were doing well. They had Apgar scores (a way to score newborn vital statistics on a scale of 1 to 10) of 8 and 9. Zachary had been moved to the NICU because he had difficulty breathing. He received a treatment of antibiotics. I have since learned that it's not uncommon for C-section babies to have difficulty breathing because there is no opportunity for the baby to clear his lungs as he descends through the birth canal. Andreas was also moved to the NICU because his brother was there and was started on a course of prophylactic antibiotics. The logic, although only explained after the fact, was because the boys shared the same environment (my uterus), they were treated the same.

Andreas was not manifesting any symptoms. Although I was only a few floors down from the NICU at the hospital, no one told me that they were starting Andreas on a course of antibiotics. The first I heard of this "treatment" was when a nurse came to inform me that Andreas had started to seize and to present me with a consent form that would allow Andreas's doctors to perform a spinal tap on him. I remember the morning like it was yesterday because it was the morning that my life took a sharp turn.

I called my husband to tell him that Andreas had seized. He thought I had confused the names: "Andreas? Don't you mean Zachary?"

Zachary shortly moved into my room at the hospital and then, after five days, he and I went home. Andreas, on the other hand, ended up staying in the hospital for five weeks. The doctors did every test imaginable on him and discovered nothing to explain the seizures. They tested him for rare genetic diseases, and they prepared us for the worst possible outcomes. No one, during all those tests, ever mentioned cerebral palsy. The label "cerebral palsy," while unknown to me at the time, would have been a lot less scary than what the doctors prepared us for.

Meanwhile, Andreas continued to seize. He was placed on anticonvulsive drugs and slept for most of those five weeks in the hospital. He continued to gain weight and grow. In fact, Andreas was gaining weight so rapidly—he was a good eater with a strong suck—that the staff would frequently recheck his weight to be sure the scale was accurate. There was a severe disconnect because the doctors were telling us that Andreas may be very sick. In fact, they said he may die. Yet, as we looked at Andreas, he looked like the picture of health.

Andreas was fine at birth, and thereafter, he continued to thrive. He began to seize after he was given three different types of prophylactic antibiotics in four doses during his first two days of life. I don't know if the drugs caused the seizures. The doctors who I've talked to about this have explained their drug protocol as a categorical good and have refused to entertain the notion that the drugs may have been a contributing factor. In fact, lawyers that I have spoken to about the situation state that they could make a better argument if Andreas had not been given drugs and something bad had happened. This fact probably supports why he was given drugs in the first place.

Since then, however, I have consulted some texts that doctors would be exposed to. In *Avery's Disease of the Newborn*, for instance, the authors state that doctors should wait and see whether a neonate develops symptoms before treating him or her with antibiotics, rather than giving the medication prophylactically (Taeusch, Ballard, and Gleason 2004). Andreas had already been moved to the neonatal intensive care unit so that he could be with his brother. He was already being watched and monitored closely.

My contention is that Andreas may have suffered an injury in utero because he was in the subordinate position in relation to his twin brother. The administration of the prophylactic antibiotics provided the second assault on his system. The combination of the two may have been too much for his system to handle.

Despite my morning sickness, the boys were large at birth. Zachary weighed seven pounds eleven ounces, and Andreas weighed six pounds two ounces. I went to term with the pregnancy and had an elective caesarean section at thirty-eight weeks. At the time, I weighed two hundred twenty-five pounds, and the boys had shown no signs of initiating their birth. Zachary was in the correct birthing position, but Andreas was horizontally oblique (on an angle across) and in the breech position.

My ob-gyn had never really considered a natural delivery, and I did not push for one. I think that she humored me as Chris and I dutifully attended Bradley classes and I wrote my birthing plan. We asked for no inoculations to be given at birth, but I did not think to instruct that no prophylactic antibiotics be administered as well. My boys were well according to the many sonograms I was instructed to have, I had gone to term, and I knew that they were very large babies for twins. I thought that I had nothing to worry about. I believe that, even if I had included a stipulation about prophylactic antibiotics, no one would have paid much attention to my instructions. As I read the hospital records after, I also saw that the boys were prepared for circumcision. On the birth plan, this was something that we stated that we did not want. Thankfully, someone must have read the document and intervened. The boys were not circumcised.

After Andreas began to seize, the head of the NICU at the hospital asked our ob-gyn if I had taken recreational drugs while pregnant. I know this happened because my ob-gyn told me that the doctor asked this question more than once. I felt like I was in a surreal universe that subscribed to inverse logic. I had taken no drugs (recreational, over-the-counter, or prescribed) while pregnant. The doctors, on the other hand, had given Andreas drugs, and when he started to inexplicably seize, they looked to see if I was the cause of the problem.

People choose labels that best suit their agenda and their vision of reality. If a mother takes recreational drugs while pregnant (which I did not), we call it reckless endangerment of the fetus. If the mother takes drugs that her physician prescribes (which I did not) and the outcome is bad, we call it unfortunate and unintended. If a physician gives drugs to a well baby who is manifesting no symptoms, we call it exercising precaution.

I made the mistake of sleeping in my room at the hospital and leaving the babies in the NICU. I did not know that the doctors could give a well baby medication without my consent and/or knowledge. I learned the hard way. I don't know with certainty that a reaction to the antibiotics caused the seizures.

The umbilical cord was wrapped around Andreas, and some doctors point to this as the potential cause of the problem. I counter that if Andreas were deprived of oxygen in utero, he would have been in distress at the time of birth, and he was not. The only other explanation I have come up with is this: Perhaps the injury occurred at some point during the gestation period and corrected itself before birth. The MRIs performed while Andreas was in the NICU showed no damage. Subsequently, I have heard two explanations for the MRI results. One physician said that the damage is so subtle that it does not show on the MRI. This explanation does not make sense to me because of the severity of Andreas's disability. Another physician explained that the tracts are not fully laid down in a baby's brain so that the place of injury does not show on an MRI. This explanation makes more sense to me.

I could only find one doctor who suggested that the antibiotics could have set off an allergic or autoimmune disorder, thereby triggering the seizures. For most doctors, antibiotics, prophylactic or otherwise, are seen as a categorical good. They will not entertain the notion that the antibiotics could have created the problem. To do so, it seems, would be to go very strongly against what they know to be true—their belief system. I am Andreas's mother, and giving drugs to a healthy newborn goes against my belief system. If I have one piece of advice to mothers, it would be this: Do not leave your baby unattended at the hospital. If possible, designate someone who will stay with the baby should the baby not be able to be in the room with you. That person should know what is being given to the baby and he or she should know what may be legally refused.

When Andreas was one year old, during our well baby visit, our pediatrician suggested that he had cerebral palsy. He was already receiving therapies through Early Intervention. Early Intervention is a wonderful program that is offered to every baby who spends time in the NICU. The program offers a wide array of home-based therapies for babies from zero to three years. Thankfully, the social worker at the hospital told me about the program. My husband did not want Andreas to be evaluated because he was concerned about Andreas being labeled, and thereby, stigmatized. I called to have him evaluated anyway. Andreas did qualify for therapies because he had torticollis— his neck was twisted to one side, causing him to hold his head abnormally—and developmental delays. When Dr. Eisenberg mentioned cerebral palsy, I told him that Andreas had not been deprived of oxygen at birth and that my working definition of cerebral palsy necessitated oxygen deprivation as its cause. Dr. Eisenberg stated that I didn't know about Andreas's oxygen supply in utero. She was right; I didn't know if the wrapped umbilical cord had prevented Andreas from getting sufficient oxygen. I also didn't know if he had been deprived of oxygen at some critical point in the gestation period; if this deprivation had been relieved by the time of birth and he was getting sufficient oxygen, that would explain why he was not in distress.

There are many questions that I do not have definitive answers for, and I have made peace with the fact that I may never know all the answers. The label "cerebral palsy" is, itself, problematic. Some people describe the label as a catch-all phrase that can mean anything. If a label can mean anything, it has no real meaning. As one mother put it, "If the label of cerebral palsy gets my child services, then I use it. Other than that, I do not use it."

Some doctors have told me that they define cerebral palsy strictly, using the label only when a deprivation of oxygen occurred at the time of birth. According to that definition,

Andreas does not have cerebral palsy. If he was deprived of oxygen before birth, then the diagnosis should be different. I do not yet have a diagnosis that is a better fit.

Some doctors I have consulted state that if a baby is not oxygen deprived at birth, he or she does not have cerebral palsy. Other doctors define cerebral palsy as oxygen deprivation either in utero or during birth. Other doctors, Dr. Bernard for instance (a gastroenterologist we consulted), merely see every disorder that the child is manifesting as a byproduct of the primary diagnosis. I would say that the primary diagnosis, then, is blocking Dr. Bernard from seeing the other issues. These are seen as secondary symptoms explained away by the primary diagnosis.

Labels powerfully shape perception. Research has proven that the label I place on someone or something powerfully shapes the perception of both the person I have labeled and anyone else who knows about the label. Academicians Robert Rosenthal and Lenore Jacobson first showed how teachers' expectations affect their students. Rosenthal and Jacobson gave teachers a roster of students and told them that some students were intellectually gifted while others where intellectually challenged. At the conclusion of the experiment, the students fell into the categories that the researchers had randomly assigned to them. The experiment, sometimes called the Pygmalion effect or Rosenthal effect, speaks to the tremendous power of perception to shape reality, demonstrating how biased expectations can affect reality and create self-fulfilling prophecies.

The researchers stated that the expectations on the part of the teachers alone created the outcome (Rosenthal and Jacobson 1992).

I have always maintained that the label "cerebral palsy" does not fit Andreas, but I have no label that suits him better. As I noted previously, Dr. Phillips did suggest that Andreas may have Angelman syndrome or, as it is unfortunately referred to in some literature, "happy puppet syndrome." When I researched Angelman, it did seem to fit Andreas. I even saw a picture of a boy carrying the diagnosis who looked identical to Andreas. Andreas has a very happy disposition, and this is one of the defining features of AS, but as Andreas's therapists explained, Andreas's disposition is situational and not frozen like an Angelman child. We did have Andreas genetically tested before his therapists shared with me this nuance of the label. Andreas, thankfully, has not tested positive for a genetic disorder.

My journey—my search for an alternative diagnosis—has led from Angelman to autism. My research on the Internet led me to a researcher. Dr. Hermit and I exchanged e-mails and had one phone conference. I had told him that I was trying to research disorders that may mimic as cerebral palsy. He told me that he would speak to his colleagues and e-mail me with a referral. He did. The referral was for Dr. Charo. I booked the appointment and felt optimistic about consulting with someone who could see through a finer lens.

Unfortunately, my confidence did wane when we arrived for our appointment. The office was dark, dirty, and unwelcoming. The doctor was running late. After we waited for an hour and a half beyond our scheduled time, the secretary convinced us to go for a cup of coffee and return.

"The doctor can help you," she said.

Previous to our appointment, Dr. Charo had faxed me a six-page questionnaire, which I'd completed and faxed back.

When we did return to the office after our coffee, the doctor had returned. It was clear from the nature of her questions that she seemed not to have read my responses that I faxed to her. In fact when we arrived for the appointment, the secretary could not locate my questionnaire and took my copy that I had brought with me.

The doctor asked me questions about Andreas but looked at what she was writing instead of looking at Andreas. She had her back to him as she went over questions that were covered in the questionnaire. I kept wishing that she would lift her eyes off the paper, turn her chair around, and look at him. When she finally did turn her attention to Andreas, she said that he looked like he had hypotonia (a state of having deficient muscle tone or tension). I felt myself grow angry; our son was now six years old. We were not the parents of a newborn suspecting that there was something wrong with their child. I had heard the word since he came home from the hospital—along with words like tone and spasticity—which unfortunately had now become part of my regular vocabulary. I was further annoyed because my husband, for reasons I couldn't imagine, asked her to define hypotonia. My blood began to boil. I didn't want to use this time to have the doctor explain basic terms. I had spent a significant amount of time conducting my own research and trying to educate myself. I had come to see Dr. Charo because I thought that she had the expertise that I needed. I wanted someone to problem solve. If this was not cerebral palsy, what could it be? To meet my expectations, my new partner on this journey would need to be very smart but also able to see Andreas and generate ideas about potential diagnoses.

The meeting with Dr. Charo went from bad to worse. I had told her that Andreas was given prophylactic antibiotics in the

NICU and that I would have never agreed to this protocol for a well newborn. Dr. Charo told me, "You cannot say that. You do not know how you would have responded."

I became angry and I showed it. "Do not tell me how I would have or I would not have responded," I retorted. I knew that anger had been building—from having to wait, from viewing Dr. Charo's disregard for the questionnaire and her refusal to look at Andreas, and from hearing a diagnosis that told me nothing and my husband asking for clarification for a basic term.

During the visit, Dr. Charo suggested that Andreas could have pyruvate dehydrogenase deficiency (PDH). She said that to test for this disease, a doctor would take an arterial blood sample and a skin graft and perform a spinal tap. She said that we could check Andreas into the hospital so that he could be sedated, and the tests could all be performed at one time. She sounded matter of fact about the procedure. She seemed to be placing a great deal of her diagnosis on Andreas's lactic acid levels from his neonatal records that I had brought with me. I was not very enthusiastic about Andreas having to go through such invasive procedures again, and I needed Dr. Charo to provide more support for her theory before I would subject him to such painful diagnostic procedures.

When we returned home, I spent five hours on the internet researching PDH. I also reread all of the documentation from Andreas's NICU records. I had discovered that the number (showing Andreas's lactic acid levels) that Dr. Charo was relying upon had been written in error; Andreas had been retested while in the hospital. I also discovered that PDH had been considered and dismissed by Andreas's doctors while he was in the NICU. I set out to get in touch with the doctors who had ordered and interpreted these tests six years ago. The neurologist, Dr. Wellby, was as unhelpful as he had been six years ago. The geneticist, Dr. Pappas at NYU, was kind and concerned. He and I spent a long time on the telephone, and in preparation for our talk, he had accessed and read Andreas's medical records. I asked Dr. Pappas if PDH had been considered and dismissed six years ago, could Andreas have PDH now. He informed me that Andreas could have PDH now even though it had been discounted when he was a newborn.

I called Dr. Charo to inform her of what I had uncovered and to ask follow-up questions. Her secretary asked me about the nature of my call. I had just spent several hours attempting to bring myself up to speed on PDH; shouldn't a follow-up call to a specialist be considered usual rather than something that I needed to explain? Even more remarkable to me, Dr. Charo was not interested in the record I'd uncovered. She did not want to talk to the geneticist who had offered so much help, she did not want to see how the lactic acid numbers had changed, and she was not interested to know what had made the doctors rule out PDH. She simply contended that even if Andreas did not have PDH then, he may have it now. Her lack of intellectual curiosity scared me.

Lastly, I asked her about her diagnosis of autism, another note she'd made on Andreas's report.

She simply replied, "I wrote that because I think he is autistic."

This felt like the tautology that exhausted parents offer their children. The child asks: "Why do I have to go to bed?" The exhausted parent answers: "Because you have to go to bed."

I decided not to have Andreas tested for PDH. I didn't have much faith or trust in this doctor to begin with, and if she could so casually label him autistic, why would I think she may be right about his having PDH? Andreas did not seem to have autism. He was nonverbal but extremely expressive nonverbally. He was highly social and supremely affectionate. I didn't trust Dr. Charo's ability to diagnose Andreas because she never really looked at him during the examination. As I've navigated the medical culture, I've discovered this tool for discernment: If the doctor does not see Andreas, I do not put much stock in his or her words. In this case, Dr. Charo, literally, did not look at Andreas. She occasionally glanced at him, but she never looked at him with her full attention. She also never spoke to him. She took notes and occasionally glanced at him as he sat to her right on his father's lap. I think that every parent wishes that his or her child would be seen. This was, I think, the intention behind the shift in our language from "disabled child" to "child with disabilities." The aim is to see the child first.

In searching out more suitable labels to cerebral palsy, I have not gotten very far. Dr. Phillips diagnosed Andreas with Angelman syndrome, and Dr. Charo diagnosed him with autism. Both turned out to be wrong, but Dr. Phillips's diagnosis seemed to be more genuine. I have since learned that another mother in the community received exactly the same diagnosis— PDH and autism—for her child from Dr. Charo. The diagnosis was not correct for this other child. When Andreas's physical therapist, Aileen, an aquatic therapist who had worked with Andreas for four years and who treated many disabled children in the community, learned of this coincidence, she asked, "Does this doctor have a cookie cutter diagnosis that she uses on all children?" This doctor heads up pediatric neurology for one of the most prestigious teaching hospitals.

Dr. Charo works at a hospital that has an fMRI machine, and that was one reason I was hopeful about seeing her. In my research, I had noticed that much of the research on functional MRIs had come out of this facility. In fact, I had called the hospital to ask how I could schedule an fMRI before we saw Dr. Charo. The hospital would not permit me to schedule a test since we had not yet seen one of their doctors. I explained that I had prescriptions for an fMRI from Andreas's neurologist and pediatrician as well as a pre-certification number from the insurance company. The woman in the radiology office would not hear of it.

When we were in Dr. Charo's office, I asked her about an fMRI. She told me that they did not use functional MRIs on children and they did not use them for diagnoses. The final ironic twist in the story of Dr. Charo is that the reason why I was interested in seeing Dr. Charo was because of her affiliation. In the end, Dr. Charo's written report made it seem that an MRI was her idea, and I was resistant. In her report, Dr. Charo noted that an MRI would be warranted but "this would entail sedation, to which the mother is opposed."

Chapter 4
Acting Unilaterally or
"Why Wasn't I Told?"

Disconnected from the Parent

In the previous chapter, I described how doctors administered antibiotics to Andreas without my knowledge or consent. I didn't think to ask about this prior to being admitted to the hospital. I had thought that doctors needed to tell parents about procedures and/or drugs before giving them to a newborn baby. I was wrong.

Sometimes we do not know what questions to ask until after an experience, and then we realize through retrospect the gaps in our knowledge. I am stunned by the questions I did not ask. Anyone who goes through in vitro fertilization should look up the rate of disability among multiple births. Multiple births carry a 50 percent chance of resulting in one or more babies with a disability. We went through four in vitro fertilization cycles, and no one ever mentioned this statistic. I never asked, and they never told. The doctors working in in vitro fertilization clinics are working on the laws of probabilities—the more eggs a woman transfers, the greater chance she has of becoming pregnant.

Looking back, I see that the medical professionals I had trusted had purposely withheld some of the information from me. I believe they did so because I wouldn't have been able to do anything about the information. I still believe in full disclosure; I still believe that I should have been told. I should have been told that, as the pregnancy progressed, the umbilical cord continued to wrap around Andreas three times. I should have been told that babies who have seizures in the NICU have a greater propensity of having cerebral palsy. I should have been told that the anticonvulsive drugs that Andreas was given themselves cause developmental delays. I would not have been able to do anything differently if I had known these pieces of information, but I do not think that doctors should have the authority to keep information from me.

Now I know that if don't ask the right questions, I won't get the information I need. I take notes during all doctor visits, and I write down questions that I wish to ask. I try to do my homework before the doctor visit so that I don't end up using valuable time to ask questions that I could easily have researched on my own. I now see that it is my job to research everything. I cannot count on anyone giving me all the information that I need to make decisions. I think that I have learned a valuable lesson. I wish that I could have learned it a different way, but this is the way it is. Sometimes if you have no knowledge of a topic—any topic— you don't know what you don't know. Medical knowledge is no different from other kinds of knowledge. For instance, I didn't know that doctors could begin a newborn on antibiotics when the baby was not manifesting any symptoms. I also didn't know that they could begin a course of drugs without at least informing the parents. I didn't know because I'd had no experience.

I find myself in a precarious position; of course, I'm not saying that, should my son require immediate lifesaving techniques and/or drugs, doctors should have to wait to tell me before acting. However, Andreas was not in a life-or-death situation, so I think that I, as his mother, should have at least been informed.

I believe that informing the mother seems to go against a culture that sees doctors as acting unilaterally. As a parent, I see this as a culture clash because whatever decision doctors make on behalf of my son, I need to live with the consequences of their decisions, and they do not.

This culture clash was recently the topic of an article in the *New York Times* written by Rahul K. Parikh, MD (Parikh 2008). In "Showing the Patient the Door Permanently," Dr. Parikh talks about deciding to fire his patient because he simply could not deal with the patient's mother. He experienced the mother as suspicious and hostile. In the entire article, Dr. Parikh never considered that the mother's suspicion and hostility may have been grounded in her own experience. In other words, he never considered that her suspicion and hostility may have been legitimate.

Within the literature written mostly by mothers, a common refrain laments encountering communication problems between mother and physician. One example comes from Patricia Stacey in *The Boy who Loved Windows*. She writes:

> When the doctor entered, I was surprised that he was fluent in English. For some reason, I had remembered him as having a thick accent. Yet when he began

speaking, I realized why I'd made the mistake; he was hard to talk to. Our words seemed to hover just in front of him and fall away. He didn't answer a question he didn't like, or he mumbled an answer, vague and dismissive. (Stacey 2004)

In the *Times* article, Dr. Parikh is asking himself the question: Is it ever morally correct to fire a patient? He never took on the bigger question of asking himself whether he was incorrectly interpreting a questioning mother as hostile and suspicious. Instead, because he saw himself as acting unilaterally, he saw himself as acting in the best interest of his patient. He never considered that the mother, too, was acting in the best interest of her son. He did not see that there are multiple visions of reality, and what really was going on with the mother was a power play. He disagreed with her, and he wanted her to keep quiet. Dr. Parikh states: "I considered my options. I could be stoic, do my job and keep the boy in my practice. I could call his mother and ask her to keep her opinions to herself so that I could focus on her son, though my instincts told me that this wouldn't stop her."

Toward the end of the article, he states that he cannot understand her reluctance regarding vaccinations. Of course he cannot understand her reluctance because he never sees her as credible. He simply takes the moral high road, and, I think, intellectually ducks the controversy concerning vaccinations, when he states, "Prevention is in my DNA. If I accepted her view, I'd be compromising."

There are, of course, exceptions to the cultural rule. Most doctors acquire their knowledge of their culture when they are medical students. A tenet of the medical culture, it seems, is this kind of unilateral thinking and acting. The NICU doctors never told our ob-gyn that they were starting Andreas on a course of prophylactic antibiotics. Doctors seem to have jurisdictions. Once my babies were born, they were under the care and jurisdiction of the NICU doctors. My ob-gyn was not kept informed about protocols and treatments of the babies, so therefore, I was not informed either.

When I think back on my pregnancy, I remember that I was considered a high-risk pregnancy because I was older and because I was carrying twins. I was asked to go for more sonograms than I care to recall. I did not ask that all of the findings of these tests be shared with me. I now realize that as I was subjecting myself and my babies to all kinds of prenatal tests, I should have asked that all the findings be shared with me. At the time, I was content to know that the babies were fine and growing and developing as they should.

When I later reviewed all of my prenatal records while writing this book, I see that each time I went for an extensive sonogram, it showed that the cord was wrapping around Andreas's (twin B) neck and foot. I don't know if the cord wrapping resulted in Andreas's injury; nor do I know if there was anything that we could have done about it. All I know is that I was never told.

I was also never told about the high rate of disabilities connected with multiple births, although it is well documented in the literature. In the course of pursuing IVF treatments, my husband and I went to four different infertility doctors and completed four IVF cycles. In all of that time, no one mentioned the issue of disability. Had I known then what I know now, I would never have transferred more than one egg at a time. During the cycle when the twins were conceived, we transferred three eggs because, as the doctor said, "Three is the gold standard." In the course of writing this book, I have discovered that the "gold standard" within medicine refers to a diagnostic test or benchmark that is regarded as definitive. It is a hypothetical ideal, and in practice, there are no ideal "gold standard" tests. I did not know enough at the time to ask how this "gold standard" impacts gestation. For instance, if all three eggs were to attach, what were the statistical predictions that one or more of the babies would have disabilities? If I had it to do over, I would transfer one egg at a time and freeze the others. I know that disabilities also arise in single births, but the statistics are much more favorable.

I know that I will never have answers to the questions surrounding what went wrong for Andreas and when it occurred. I have no other choice but to accept that I do not know and move on. I try to create something good from my experience and let this experience inform my current choices so that I do not make the same errors again. I wish that when doctors were treating children with disabilities, they would understand how former experiences with the medical culture have shaped the people who stand before them now.

When I reflect on all the times when I, as the mother, was not given a piece of useful information, I see that there were times when having the knowledge would have made a significant difference and times when it would have made no difference at all. I can think of two times where it would have made a significant difference. First, as I've noted, I would never have put back more than one egg at a time during an in vitro fertilization cycle had I known about the risks of disability regarding multiples. Conceiving twins during a spontaneous pregnancy would have been a different story, but I had options.

The other time when having knowledge would have made a difference was when Andreas was in the NICU and given prophylactic antibiotics. I would not have agreed, had I been given the choice, to give a baby who was presenting no symptoms drugs. Having knowledge of some of the other developments in Andreas's case would have made no difference, but it would have been good to know exactly what was going on. It would have been good to know that Andreas most likely had cerebral palsy while he was an infant. In retrospect, his cerebral palsy was obvious, but no one ever mentioned it was a possibility. It would have been good to know that anticonvulsive drugs cause learning delays. Knowing this would not have changed what happened, but I should have been told anyway.

In other circumstances, I wasn't told about potential risks, but in these cases, I did not follow the doctor's orders because I had done my own research. For instance, I did not give Andreas mineral oil when the gastroenterologist recommended doing so because I'd learned about the risks associated with using it. Similarly, I did not give him melatonin to help him sleep even though the geneticist endorsed it. I did not place Andreas under the sleep-deprived condition the neurologist suggested before taking him for an EEG. In fact, I never had the test performed at all. I knew that he was not seizing, and I did not need a test to confirm what I already knew.

I'm not trying to buck the system. I'm just trying to take care of my son in the best way that I know how. Given that the medical system is highly specialized, there is no longer a generalist overlooking the whole spectrum of medicine with the welfare of the individual in mind. Given the current state of medicine, I feel that I need to be the gatekeeper.

Chapter 5
Constructing Mom as Obstacle
or "Mother Refuses"

Disconnected from Alternative Points of View

In the previous chapter, I discussed an article written by a physician who could not tolerate the patient's mother. He experienced her as resistant. I think there is a perception at play within the medical culture that sees mothers as the obstacle to healing. There are, of course, doctors who see the mother and doctor in a partnership, but these doctors are rare. I think those doctors who create a collaborative relationship go against the medical culture. It is my contention that doctors learn this negative perception of mothers from the way doctors speak about mothers. In the previously mentioned article, the physician refers to the patient's mother as "this lady." The way he refers to the mother sounds dismissive at best. All those who are a part of a particular culture are indoctrinated in the beliefs of that culture. This is why doctors who themselves are mothers may also acquire the negative perceptions of mothers. It is part of the cultural knowledge.

My theory is that it is the rare doctor who sees mothers as people of wisdom and from whom occasionally the doctor may learn. Previously, I discussed how language shapes perception. I know of many mothers of children with disabilities who went against the conventional wisdom of the doctor. By following a protocol that the mother selected, the child improved. We have all heard of families who simply refuse to accept the doctor's prognoses for their children. There are many testimonials from families who have children who are walking, talking, and graduating from school who doctors believed would not be capable of any of these milestones.

We all play a role in creating this aspect of the medical culture. We, too, do not speak of the mother as the authority of her child's health. We recreate and reinforce the myth that doctors know our children better than their mothers do. The lingering myth is that mothers are too connected emotionally to have any judgment with regard to her child. I think we have it wrong. It is precisely because we are so emotionally connected that we have the capacity for insight. Many mothers are driven to research and follow protocols because of the love that they have for their children.

At times, the research that a mother has done produces a hostile reaction in her child's doctor. I think that this is because, once you have educated yourself, you begin to ask questions, and you may refuse to do what you are told. In my experience, not all doctors embrace questions, and many health care professionals dislike it when you do not obey. For example, I recall a doctor's visit when Andreas was not feeling well. We arrived at the pediatrician's office and were shown into the examination room. Andreas was snuggled into my chest when the nurse came in and told me, "Take off his clothes so that I can weigh him." I told the nurse that weighing him was not necessary since he was eating and drinking. I knew that he had not lost weight, and I knew that he was not dehydrated. The nurse grew visibly annoyed. She said that the circumstances did not matter, and it was procedure to weigh all the children who come into the office. I told her that I understood and that I would explain to the doctor why Andreas was not weighed that day. When the doctor did arrive, and I explained my reasoning, it was a nonissue.

I provide the example of office procedure because I think that the procedure is frequently used to steamroll mothers into compliance. For instance, I could never understand the procedure of tying an infant to a table to give him or her an injection. I never did it, and I used to watch infants screaming in the doctor's office as the parent helplessly looked on.

I have heard testimony from smart mothers who questioned their pediatricians and were then conciliatory in the face of the doctor's reactions. One of Andreas's therapists told me about questioning her pediatrician regarding the vaccination schedule for her children. She told me that the doctor made her feel stupid for questioning the efficacy of the protocol. The therapist told me that she felt embarrassed and accepted the vaccinations as the doctor had prescribed. It is difficult to respond like an adult when someone in the medical culture addresses you as a child, but acquiescence confirms the impression the offending speaker has created.

In my teaching, I offer my students the concept of the perception check. It is a way to call someone you're interacting with on her or his behavior without resorting to blame. As you have read of my encounters with some doctors, I do not always follow my own advice. Sometimes I forget and I react. I tell my students that it is always better to form a response (which implies thinking about one's options and the effectiveness of each option) rather than blurting out a reaction. I know from personal experience, when I have been able to do it, that the perception check can be very powerful. In this context, a perception check would sound like this: "The way you just spoke to me sounded like how one might speak to a child. Did you intend to dismiss my question? Are you impatient with your patients asking you questions? Did I catch you at a bad time?" These questions redirect the conversation back to the doctor and create the message that you are not accepting the condescension. You, as the speaker, are asking the doctor to begin to engage with you as an adult without blaming him or her.

The medical culture would greatly be improved if doctors learned to discern the intention of a mother's objection. Every objection is different, and it is important to learn the motivation behind each. Some people object for the sake of objecting, and the objection is rooted in a power play. Some people object because they do not understand, and they, therefore, need to be educated. Some people object because they have some information that the other does not have. The appropriate response, then, is to listen. Communication experts have been pointing out the importance of understanding a person's motives for time untold. Allow me to recast this simple concept in the context of the medical community; doctors need to listen to their patients in order to understand the patients' intentions and the reasoning at work. On one side of the communication transaction, it is important for the parents to listen to the intention of the doctor, and on the other end of the communication transaction, it is important for the doctor to listen to the intention of the parent. Sometimes this is easy to do, and sometimes it's not. It requires that both parties pay attention to *how* something is said and not only *what* is said.

Sometimes, how something is said carries the meaning of the message. For instance, I ask my students if they can hear the intention of their mothers when they complain that Mom lists all of the opportunities they would have had if they'd stayed home rather than moved away for college. Often, behind the words is the mother's fear of losing her child. Hearing someone else's intentions doesn't necessarily require you to make grand changes—the child doesn't have to move back home, for example—but it facilitates greater understanding.

How you speak to the person with whom you're communicating is generally shaped by how you see him or her. I could speak about how I think that I'm perceived during office visits, but for the most accurate representation, I think that it's better if I present the doctors' own language from their medical reports. The first report that I'll quote comes from the geneticist that we consulted to determine whether Andreas tested positive for Angelman syndrome. The doctors wrote, "There is an ill defined history of possible infection/sepsis that the mother does not agree with."

This statement is a distortion, and it is misleading. The geneticist made it seem that the NICU doctors thought Andreas was septic and I disagreed with them. How could I disagree with a doctor's diagnosis of sepsis? This was out of my area of expertise. The NICU doctors, however, never suspected Andreas of sepsis; they suspected Zachary of sepsis. It seemed like the geneticists latched onto the idea that I disagreed without understanding the nature of my disagreement. I disagreed with the protocol of giving antibiotics to a well baby who was not manifesting any symptoms because they suspected his twin brother of having sepsis. I did not follow the logic of such a decision. Would the doctors, for instance, have given prophylactic anticonvulsives to Zachary if his twin brother, Andreas, had suffered from seizures at birth? Would the same logic—that the boys had shared the same environment, my uterus—be acceptable in this circumstance? Neither child, as it turned out, was septic.

For another example, I return to the pediatric neurologist that we consulted in the hope that she would give us insight from her specialization of diseases mimicking as cerebral palsy. The doctor wrote up her suggestion that Andreas may have pyruvate dehydrogenase deficiency and stated that the parents were not amenable to the tests she recommended. She omitted our reasons for our lack of amenability. She does not state that the neonatal lactic acid test had been redone in the NICU and had resulted in different levels. She did not say that the parents didn't have much confidence in her diagnosis as she was uninterested in reading the patient's complete medical history. She did not mention that since she had also diagnosed Andreas with autism, the parents were skeptical about subjecting their son to a series of intrusive tests to be conducted by someone they did not see as credible.

The word Dr. Charo used in the report was *amenable*. Amenable means willing to follow advice or suggestion; tractable; submissive. Amenable means responsible to authority. The etymology of the word is Latin, and it means to lead, as in to drive cattle or to shout out or to threaten. The doctor's word choice was dead on since we were not amenable, but she failed to mention any reason for our lack of amenability. She simply stated, "From a diagnostic perspective he [Andreas] would merit a full neurometabolic evaluation if the parents were amenable, which does not appear to be the case."

Dr. Charo's report suggested that we were acting contrary to her wishes for the sake of being contrary. Toward the end of the report, she stated that the tests that she was recommending "would entail sedation, to which mother is opposed." She did not say that I didn't agree because I didn't have any confidence in her diagnosis. There is never any mention as to why the mother was opposed. Sometimes, when trying to make sense of messages, one needs to look at what is not said in addition to what is said.

The medical culture frequently constrains the range of acceptable emotions from mothers. In preparation for this book, I reread Andreas's medical records from the NICU. I read all the notes from the medical staff; often they had recorded things like "mother distraught," "mother teary," or "mother upset." They also added "provided support."

Another mother, Miriam Edelson, in *My Journey with Jake: A Memoir of Parenting and Disability*, offers a similar sentiment about her experience with the hospital staff while her son was in and out of hospitals as a baby. Edelson writes:

> I try to remain composed. It is hard enough to get information around here—especially from anyone in authority—without me showing signs of cracking when it comes. I've learned something in two months here; any attitude other than gratitude is frowned upon. A mother's emotion, particularly anger, is often dismissed as hysteria. (Edelson 2000)

Environments also create their own kind of discourse, and interiors can be seen as forms of nonverbal communication. My experience at the time of the births was exacerbated by the environment of the NICU. The message created by NICU at the hospital where I delivered the boys was not a positive one.

It seemed like those who created the NICU never gave much thought as to how the environment would impact the babies and the parents who would be spending a lot of time there.

I had just given birth to twins; Zachary was home with our nanny while Andreas stayed in the hospital. Andreas slept most days because he was heavily sedated with anticonvulsive medication. I was recovering from major surgery, and instead of bed rest, I was commuting into Manhattan every day to take my place by Andreas's isolette. I watched as Andreas was poked and prodded continuously and was subjected to more tests than I have had in a lifetime. He lived within an environment, the NICU, which I could only imagine as jarring to a newborn's sensibilities. As an adult, my nerves would be frazzled after putting in eight-hour days in the NICU. It was bright, the music that was on the radio suited the tastes of the nurses, and the nurses would yell to each other from across the room. One day, I counted that the steel medical charts were dropped three times onto bare linoleum floors. Added to these noises were the (necessary) continuous beeps of equipment. The quality of life in a NICU is appalling, so yes, I think, the mother has good reason to be upset.

The other reason why these notes unnerve me is because, when you spend time in the NICU or the hospital, there is no privacy. You are out in the open, and every emotion that you, as a mother, experience is on display. And still, the mother frequently feels straitjacketed by what is considered an acceptable emotion. As Edelson puts it, "There is nowhere to hide in a hospital; even the bathroom is not a private place" (Edelson 2000).

After giving birth, I most craved private time with my family. I wanted to rest, recover, and bond with my children. This was something else we all had to sacrifice because of circumstances. To make matters worse, the doctors were asking if I was responsible for Andreas's condition. I was under their unilateral authority when it came to every invasive test and procedure. I wish that the medical culture had some sensitivity to all of these factors when they were dealing with families. It would not change the circumstances, but it would bring a very much-needed human touch to administering to families.

Chapter 6
The Language of Contradiction
or "Catch-22"

Disconnected from Alternate Logic in the Hospital Setting

Several examples of contradiction in language, or catch-22, come to mind. I'll share one I experienced in a hospital setting and another that comes from a school setting.

After Dr. Phillips suggested that Andreas may have Angelman syndrome, we took him to a geneticist at a top teaching hospital in New York. After the clinician drew blood, a doctor from the hospital called and told me that they would need to redraw for the mirodelition array genetic test. I asked why, and she said that she didn't know. I wondered how a doctor could call a mother and tell her that her child's blood needed to be redrawn without anticipating that the mother would question why. She called back and said there was not enough DNA material in the sample. This sounded suspicious since they'd taken several vials of blood. I decided that I would get the test performed elsewhere.

I suggested to Dr. Phillips that the hospital may have lost the blood sample and that the doctor who called was trying to avoid telling me. Dr. Phillips confirmed my suspicion and added that the hospital's actions were further mystifying because of mixed messages. The doctors at the New York hospital told me that they routinely send their blood samples to a hospital in Boston for analysis. I learned that the Boston hospital sends its blood samples to a hospital in Atlanta for analysis. It was clear to me that Andreas's samples had been lost.

Then the doctors' report arrived in the mail. I had requested it from Dr. Phillips, as the geneticist had not sent me a copy of the report she sent to him. The report contained twelve factual errors. There were so many errors in the report that I wrote an addendum and sent it to the neurologist and copied Andreas's pediatrician. Here's where the contradiction came into play: The geneticist never stated that the bloods were even drawn for the microdelition array test. She stated that she was recommending this test as the next step. She omitted that the reason why we went to her in the first place was to have this test performed. In addition to the errors, the report that the doctors wrote was dishonest. It differed from what the doctor had told me on the telephone. I wrote a response both to the geneticist and the director of genetics at the hospital. I never heard back from either. I did hear back from the neurologist. He left me a very generous voice mail stating that he thought my impressions were on point. I greatly appreciated getting that message.

This example of contradiction is convoluted, as are many examples of contradictory language. To sum it up, the neurologist who suggested the blood test said of the report, "It made my head hurt to try to figure out what those words meant." Maybe that was the intention of the report. The language was so confusing that it did make one's head hurt. As the reader, I had to first remember that I had gone to this hospital particularly to have this test performed. Second, I had to ask myself if it made sense that they had said there was an insufficient blood sample to do the DNA test. I am not a physician, but I know that a DNA sample could be drawn from a swab of the mouth. Third, I needed to remember both statements could not be true. It could not be true that the test was inconclusive *and* it had not been performed.

I did arrange for Andreas to have an entire series of genetic tests performed. I went to Greenwich Hospital in Connecticut and asked to speak to a manager. I was put in touch with Kathy Mitas, lab director. I explained to Kathy what had happened and the efforts I was taking to ensure that Andreas have only one more puncture. I was not going to do this again. Kathy was very kind and understanding. I wanted to have everything prepared ahead of time so that I could just show up with Andreas and the vials would be ready. Kathy was good enough to fax me the work orders for the blood samples, and when I noticed that one was wrong, she corrected it. I was very happy that Kathy was not one of the majority among the medical culture, who believe outsiders know nothing about their work and refuse to embrace mothers who want to be included. She arranged that a manager, Edmund Simon, draw Andreas's bloods. The bloods were drawn professionally using one puncture, and results came back negative for all tests.

The next example of contradictory language, or catch-22, comes from within the school setting. After Andreas attended nursery school with his brother, we placed him in a school for children with special needs. Throughout the early intervention program, Andreas's therapists were advocating that Andreas shift from receiving therapy at home to receiving facility-based therapy. I did look into this option when Andreas was very small. We went to see Dr. Hayes, the physiatrist at a special needs school, when Andreas was about one year old. Dr. Hayes agreed that Andreas should be "in program." I was on leave from my job at the time, the kids had a wonderful full-time nanny, Andreas was receiving all of his therapies at home, and he had a typically developing twin brother at home whom he could model. All of these things added up to the decision to keep him at home. Dr. Hayes did not know all of the particulars about Andreas's life because she did not ask. I didn't feel that she saw Andreas as an individual, so I never put much credence into her recommendations.

The recommendation from the physiatrist at the school for children with special needs is an example of contradiction because I knew that the circumstances of Andreas's life made home a better place to be when he was very small. Yet, I was being told—by someone who had no knowledge of his home life—that he would do better away from us. Later, I would discover that Andreas, in fact, did not do better at this school, even when he was older.

As a mother of a typically developing child and a child of special needs, I am suspicious of messages that say that what is best for special needs children differs from what is best for typically developing children. If it is best for typically developing children to be home with their caretakers, then this is also best for children with special needs. If it is not best for typically developing preschoolers to be in school all day, why would that be best for children with special needs? If it is not acceptable to place very small typically developing children on a school bus, why would it be acceptable to place a child with special needs on a school bus when he or she is very small? I am not talking about when circumstances require these choices, but rather when the family has options. I do find it contradictory that some people speak about children with special needs in a separate category from other children.

Disconnected from Alternate Logic in the School Setting

When Andreas was four years old, I enrolled him at the school for special needs children that we'd visited earlier, even though during my first tour of the school, I'd cried. I enrolled him because I did not think I had any other options. What I know now that I didn't know then is that I always have options. If I see that I don't, I'm not looking with enough imagination. I also now try to follow my first instincts. If something feels wrong, it is wrong. I now know, I hope, to walk away from that which does not feel right.

The school year turned out to be a disaster. Maybe *disaster* is too strong a word. The school offered good day care, but therapeutically and educationally, it was not up to standard. I knew from the beginning that it was not good enough, but Andreas was happy and well cared for, so I let it go. I was busy teaching and lulled myself into believing that he was getting what he needed. I knew from the start, for instance, that the speech therapist was in way over her head. Andreas is nonverbal and has very involved therapeutic needs. He was assigned one speech therapist who was supposed to do prompt therapy (hands-on therapy that assists the child in making the appropriate sounds) as well as augmentative communication (the use of devices in order to communicate). The oral motor skills (therapy which works on the motor skills of the mouth) were not addressed at all. I knew that this therapist was not capable. When I asked the therapist to try Andreas on a particular *speech generating* device, she called me to ask on what page she could find the device in the special needs catalog.

I did call the manager of speech therapy and expressed my reservations about the therapist we'd been assigned. The manager replied, "She's the best we have."

I knew that I was in trouble but unbelievably, I accepted the manager's answer. In retrospect, I now see that when someone says, "She/he/it's the best we have," it closes down potential problem solving. When you tell someone that what he or she is having a problem with is the best available, you're making the person seem perpetually dissatisfied. As the listener, that person must conclude that, if he or she isn't satisfied with the best, then he or she will never be satisfied. I think the strategy is used to end the conversation, which it did. Andreas's therapist was not the best speech therapist, and I knew it. After the conversation with the manager, I started to look at my options to place Andreas in another school.

The physical therapy and the occupational therapy at Andreas's school were not much better than the speech therapy. The physical therapy was performed by a PTA (physical therapy assistant), and the occupational therapy was performed by a CODA (occupational therapy assistant).

I informed the school district, which was now overseeing Andreas's education, about the lack of credentials of the people working with Andreas. The school district representative said, "That cannot be."

The district only saw the reports that were signed by fully-licensed therapists, but in practice, those therapists never saw Andreas. Since my husband, my nanny, and I were at the school every day, we knew that the supervisors never came upstairs to the therapy room. We never used the school bus, so we saw Andreas in his class at drop off in the morning and at pick up at the end of the day. We would also drop in during the day so we had a good basis to draw a conclusion.

It was not just the credentials and lack of expertise that bothered us about Andreas's therapists, but also the way that the therapy was delivered was substandard. There was one big room where the therapy was performed. Therapists pulled children out of their class for thirty minutes of therapy. If you deducted travel time, each session amounted to twenty minutes of therapy. Andreas is a highly social child and is very interested in watching other children. The CODA, or the person acting as his occupational therapist, thought that the other children were a distraction, so she had him do his therapy while facing a wall. She had a booming voice, and she would scream his name at him. Luckily, Andreas thought this was funny, and whenever she would yell his name, he would laugh. Andreas is an easygoing kid, so he was amenable to any situation in which he was placed.

At the end of the school year, the reports detailing Andreas's progress arrived in the mail. I carried them in my bag for two weeks—unopened. I knew that the news would not be good, so I was preparing myself before I read them. When I did read them, I was devastated. For every skill, Andreas performed at the level of an infant. I immediately thought about the incongruity between the school "therapists" and the private therapists who continued to treat Andreas. I later found out that Andreas's teachers and therapists at his school used measurement tools that are not designed for nonverbal children. By using these tools, Andreas's therapists set him up to fail.

I next met with the school's principal and Andreas's teacher. I asked them how, in good conscious, they could use a measurement tool that was not designed for Andreas. They pushed off the responsibility onto the school district, telling me that they used the measurement tools because that's what the school districts wanted them to use and that the district knew that the tools didn't give an accurate assessment of a nonverbal child. I told the principal that I saw the reports for what they were and that I know not to give much attention to them. I wondered, though, about the nonnative parent with a nonverbal child who received a report like this. His or her child may be smart but trapped in a body that could not perform and could not speak. I asked if she felt any trepidation about shaping the attitudes of those parents and influencing their expectations of their children. She did not answer me, and I assume that the school personnel are still doing what they have always done.

In the meantime, I had already begun to look around for another school. I made the mistake of not informing my school district of what was going on. It never occurred to me to tell them. I thought that, since I did not like where he was, I needed to fix it. It did not occur to me to seek their help. I knew that Andreas would not be staying where he was, but I didn't know where he'd be going.

My focus, at the time, was to get Andreas out of the school. During that meeting, the principal told me that the upcoming kindergarten class (which she was happy to have Andreas join) would consist of "low functioning" kids. As of then, she had two boys from Andreas's current class enrolled. One boy seemed to be severely autistic. The other boy was so sick and highly medicated that he slept during class most days.

According to his private therapists, Andreas was making great strides, and according to the therapists at the school, at four years old, he had the abilities of a seven- to nine-month-old. I had found a school for Andreas near where I taught that required the child to be cognitively intact, even if he was physically disabled. I knew that the reports were damaging to Andreas, so I told the school district that I wanted the reports thrown away and I was going to hire Andrea's private therapists to write reports of their own. They did and I sent the new reports to the school I was considering. The school's administrator's, at the last moment, did not accept Andreas because they said that they could not get him to respond as they wanted.

After the reports, we had to attend a meeting at Andreas's school. I sat at the table and listened as teachers and therapists spoke of all that Andreas could not accomplish. I didn't say anything but instead just listened. After they all talked about what Andreas could not do, the physiatrist said (without any sense of irony), "It doesn't matter because he's not going anywhere. He's going to be here next year, and we will continue treating him."

I think the physiatrist meant to sound supportive, but I thought what they were proposing was insane. Andreas was not able to accomplish what was asked of him, so the plan was to keep him where he was and to keep doing what was currently being done.

Just as it had gone against common sense for doctors to recommend a test that I thought they'd already performed, it went against common sense for a school to use measurement instruments that set up the student to fail. Once he did fail, it defied common sense for them to recommend that things be kept the same.

I left the school meeting determined that Andreas would not return in the fall. The school was very willing to have Andreas join the kindergarten class and to keep him "in program" while charging our home school district forty thousand dollars a year. In anticipation of his end-of-year meeting with the school district, I asked that personnel from his current school not be invited to the meeting. Instead, I asked that his private therapists take their place and speak about Andreas's true capabilities. Since we were not admitted to the school of my preference, and none of the other special schools were acceptable, I asked that the school district approve and recognize his private therapies as his school equivalent for the upcoming school year. Thankfully, the school district approved, and Andreas's private therapists have been wonderful. Andreas has happily completed his second year of customized education and will have the same program next year. He is happy, learning, and with people who see him as capable. I cannot ask for more.

During Andreas's meeting with our school district, I argued that Andreas was never given the opportunity to succeed at the special needs school. In fact, in many cases I could show how he had been set up to fail. I think that this special needs school simply used kids like Andreas. I realize that I am going out on a limb here. The school district is in the situation of needing to educate all children. The special needs school claims to the district that they can satisfy that need. I could see how many parents are just happy that their child has a school to attend. In our situation, the special school merely babysat Andreas and charged the school district handsomely for the service.

From my experience raising a child with disabilities, I drew up a list of ten experiences in which health care professionals used contradiction. I will list them for you so that you can see how insidious this language pattern is. The list of contradictions includes:

> ➢ Give a well baby prophylactic antibiotics.

> ➢ Give a seizing baby immunizations (MMR) that may cause seizures.

> ➢ Give a baby with reflux and constipation an antacid medication that may cause the body to produce more acid and can worsen constipation.

> ➢ Deprive a child who has had one seizure from sleep in preparation for an EEG.

> ➢ Recommend a test to confirm that a baby has reflux when his reflux is self-evident.

> ➢ Ask the family to complete the paperwork regarding confidentiality and then announce to the entire room full of patients the reason for your visit.

> ➢ Use measurement tools that are designed for verbal children on children who are nonverbal.

> ➢ Recommend that a child stay in a program and maintain the same treatment plan when the plan is not working.

> ➢ Refuse to hear that the diagnosis you are delivering for a patient was already considered and dismissed by other physicians.

> ➢ Diagnose a child who has made one visit to your office, during which you barely turned your chair to clinically observe the patient, with autism.

I assume that there are physicians who would challenge some of the items on my list. They would probably say that I am a novice and do not understand the reasons why these examples are not contradictions within the medical or educational culture.

Chapter 7
The Language of Ambiguity or "Deception by Ambiguity"

Disconnected from Clarity in the Hospital Setting

Ambiguity implies a choice. Some words have ambiguity built into them. The word *host*, for instance, can mean guest, enemy, or eucharist. The ambiguity of the word informs us that we can see the host as friend, foe, or godlike depending on both choice and circumstance. If, however, someone is ambiguous in order to deceive, we can interpret ambiguity differently. For instance, in the previous chapter, I wrote about the geneticist who lost Andreas's blood samples and then wrote the report using ambiguous language, seemingly, to cover up the error. The language of the report was so unclear that I wasn't sure what the doctor was saying.

The report reads as follows: "Laboratory unable to extract optimal quality of DNA for analysis. Must send repeat sample." This statement matches what I was told on the phone. However, toward the end of the report, the doctors write, "Although there is no documentation provided for chromosome analysis, microarray would be adequate." Here the doctors seem to be saying that they had no prescription for the microarray test, and they seem to suggest that the test was never done. The statement seems to contradict the earlier claim that there was not enough DNA material in the blood sample. The language was even more confusing given that the reason we went to a geneticist in the first place was because we wanted to have the microarray test performed. The report suggests that the test was the doctor's suggestion. The next sentence reads, "We have informed Andreas's parents that a repeat specimen is required in order to properly interpret results from microarray." Now the report seems to be saying that a test was performed, but the results cannot be interpreted.

I am but one mother trying to make my way in a system that is not set up to assist me. I think that my experience may be magnified by the multitudes of parents trying to make their way as well. When I mention to my husband that the geneticists' report contained twelve errors, he replied, "They must hate to write those reports."

His response was an example of one way that we maintain the status quo. This is one example of how our language may work to maintain a culture that does not serve us. Every time we make an excuse for a doctor, we are keeping things the same. An example of this is the almost knee-jerk reaction some people will give when confronted by the complaint of a cold, uncaring doctor. Some people will offer the cliché that the doctor needs emotional distance in order to do his or her job. I have never bought that argument. I would rather be treated by a doctor who cares too much any day.

The message health care providers in the assisted reproduction industry deliver concerning the risks associated with multiples is another example of ambiguity. In a recent *New York Times* article, Stephanie Saul addressed the issue. Saul contends that the industry's position is that multiples are risky because the human uterus is designed to carry one fetus at a time. At the same time, she offers that, for many doctors, "twins are not such a risky bet because most are healthy" (Saul 2009).

My boys are healthy, but one boy has a severe case of cerebral palsy. Saul points out that cerebral palsy occurs four to six times more often in twins than it does in single babies.

The industry's message is ambiguous with regard to the risks associated with multiples because they want a greater success rate, which translates into dollars. Fertility doctors state that couples who are trying to conceive are driving the practice of multiple egg transfer.

As I reflect on my four IVF cycles with four different doctors over three years, I realize it was the doctors who pushed a high number of egg transfers. At one time, we transferred seven eggs at once. The doctor came into the operating room and said, "We have twelve fertilized eggs. Take a few minutes to decide how many you want to transfer."

This experience is not in keeping with how the industry claims to speak about the question of how many eggs to transfer. Doctors state that they inform the patient of the consequences of transferring more than one egg and that patients' wishes are the driving force behind the risky practice of multiple transfers.

Over the years, not one doctor spoke about risks. *The New York Times Magazine* recently ran a front cover story featuring the headline "If Health Care is Going to Change, His Ideas Will Change it." In the article, Dr. Brent James is featured as the savior of health care. The author paraphrases James as saying that, throughout history, doctors have done more harm than good (Leonhart 2009). This failure on our doctor's part to warn my husband and me about the risks we were taking seems to me a clear example of causing harm.

Saul's article also speaks about a waiver that couples sign highlighting the risks attached with multiples. My husband and I have never heard of a waiver.

What is most striking about the doctors Saul quotes in her article is that they state that IVF is unusual within the medical community because (1) doctors are yielding to pressure from parents, (2) doctors are not following their own guidelines to transfer a single egg, and (3) doctors are giving patients the autonomy to decide how many embryos to transfer. I wonder what makes the IVF context so different from other medical contexts. For the sake of argument, let's contrast this context to the vaccination context. One, are doctors yielding to parents who object to the current vaccination schedule? Two, are doctors not yielding to aggressive guidelines? Three, are doctors giving the patients the autonomy to make their own decisions about vaccinations? The answer to all these questions is no. It seems, on the surface, that when it is economically beneficial to yield to the patient, doctors will do so regardless of the risks. In the case of vaccinations, it is economically beneficial for parents to vaccinate their children early and often. Some doctors will not entertain delaying vaccinations and/or spreading them out over more time. The message concerning vaccinations is unambiguous.

Saul's article sets up an interesting scenario. The point of the article is that doctors keep warning parents about the risks of multiples, but parents are not listening. No doctor ever warned my husband and me about risks. In fact Dr. Isak, the first fertility doctor we consulted, told us, "Put back two eggs. This way, you may get a boy and a girl. Instant family."

Saul points to the frequent refrain I've presented in this book—blame the parent. No doctor ever warned me about risks, but now they claim that I did not heed their warnings. One doctor quoted in the article, Dr. Maurizio Macaluso, who runs the CDC's women's health and fertility branch, stated it this way: "You can't convince a couple that having twins is a bad thing … That's a major communication problem" (Saul 2009). You can never convince a couple about all the risks associated with multiples if you never try or if you construct ambiguous messages.

Ambiguity means to wander around or to be unclear. Sometimes ambiguity is expected. Politicians sometimes use ambiguity as a communication strategy so that different groups will create different meanings. Some organizations, it seems, cannot help themselves. For instance, I recently received a letter from my insurance company, and both Andreas's therapist and I did not know for sure whether or not they were denying or covering benefits. However, when a doctor seems to use ambiguity to cover up a mistake, I feel particularly unsettled and distrustful. The doctor/patient relationship is different from all other relationships because of the level of need. When ambiguity is used by an insurance company, I do not take it to heart because I see my relationship with the insurance company differently than I see my relationship to my doctor. I see the insurance company as a bureaucracy that cares mostly about keeping costs down. I would like to see my doctor as someone who cares about me and my family outside of the context of money.

When I took Andreas to yet another doctor's appointment (this appointment was with a neurologist who specializes in cerebral palsy and its mimics), my husband asked: "Why do you keep going to doctors?"

I answered that I keep going because I keep hoping that I can find a decent doctor who can help.

Chapter 8
Thoughtless Language or "Thought and Action Have Parted Company"

Disconnected from Thought in the Doctor's Waiting Room

I attribute so much of the hurtful language that occurs within the medical culture to lack of thought rather than to malice. I have a group of examples that I use in the classroom to show that damage may occur when you do not intend to hurt someone's feelings but you simply are not thinking about what you are saying. We all carry memories of experiences of thoughtless speech both as receiver of these messages as well as speakers. We have also learned that once words are said, we cannot take our words back.

In class, we talk about a maxim learned as a child: Sticks and stones may break my bones but words will never hurt me. My students arrive at the awareness that the maxim is a lie, and when I ask why we repeat it, they say because parents do not want their kids hurt by words. Even though we may want to protect our children, it is inevitable that we will be hurt by others' words, and the maxim won't help. In fact, the maxim may hurt because it tells the child that he or she has no reason to feel hurt. It may even contribute to the damage occurring in the first place. It tells the child that words are not important, tacitly granting him or her permission to use hurtful words.

The medical culture is governed by routine and procedure. The damage is created when professionals follow routine and procedure without thinking. Frequently, when I call the insurance about Andreas, the representative asks me if I have permission to speak on his behalf. They are merely going by the script that they have been given and are not thinking that they are speaking to the mother of a nonverbal, seven-year-old boy.

The insurance example is more comical than serious. In a doctor's office, however, the stakes are much higher. After Andreas had one seizure after being seizure-free for several years, we arrived late in the day for an appointment with a new neurologist. It had been a grueling day after a difficult night. The woman behind the front desk was not very friendly. She continued the task of putting away office supplies as we stood at her desk waiting for her to acknowledge us. When I asked for a place to change Andreas, she motioned us toward an examination room that had not been cleaned after the previous patient. She told us, "Take your dirty diaper with you after you change him." Unfortunately, this example of thoughtlessness is common is my experience with the medical culture. I wondered why common sense and common courtesy is so uncommon within the medical culture.

What followed next during our introduction to the office was the epitome of lack of thought. I filled out the necessary paperwork, including the statement of confidentiality that the office personnel so doggedly persisted we complete, and sat down.

The receptionist began a conversation with me from across the room.

"How is he doing?" she asked.

I called back, "Fine."

"He's the one with the seizures, right?" she persisted. "Is he okay now?"

Why did I just sign those pieces of paper only to have the purpose of my visit announced to a roomful of strangers? I thought. Instead, I said nothing.

The problem is that the medical culture complies with the requirements but doesn't seem to think about what the procedures mean.

Sometimes, however, things do work for the best. The violation of our confidentiality did work to our benefit. The doctor was running late. We had a 5:00 p.m. appointment, and the receptionist told us that he was running one to two hours behind schedule. There were two families waiting ahead of us. She asked, again from across the room, how I planned on paying for the visit. I said that I did not know if I would be staying. Andreas had already had a long day. It was now his dinner time, and if we stayed, we would not get home before 9:00 p.m. It was too late for him. One very kind family in the waiting room offered their appointed time to us. Their kindness touched me.

When I approached the other mother, she said, "We've been in your circumstance. We wish you all the best."

Later in the elevator as we were leaving, we encountered the father. He was getting his daughter something to drink since they were going to be there for a while. I will always remember his simple, gracious words: "Too many people are blind and deaf to the needs of others."

It was also not lost on me that the receptionist's clumsiness was responsible for this gesture. They knew of our circumstance because it was announced.

Disconnected from Thought in the Hospital Setting

Another example of thoughtless speech occurred when Andreas was three years old and needed oral surgery. His mouth had deteriorated as a result of the combination of the medications he was on during his first year of life, a bad case of acid reflux, his habit of grinding his teeth, and our bad habit of giving him a bottle and immediately putting him to bed. He had so many cavities that his dentist suggested filling them all at once in the hospital under general anesthetic. The dentist and the hospital staff were excellent—with one exception. A nurse greeted us and brought us to the operating room. They had given us a private room to wait in so Andreas was comfortably sitting on his father's lap and watching a movie.

One of the first things the nurse said to Andreas was, "Are you going to be a big boy and walk to the operating room or are you going to be a baby and have your daddy carry you?"

I don't think that this comment was malicious. It was just that the nurse didn't think before she spoke. I ask my students to think before they open their mouths and ask themselves if their comment is more likely to hurt than help. Unfortunately, I don't think that they teach this lesson in medical school, or maybe I've just been unlucky in meeting people who did not learn it.

The nurse's comment, even if offered to a child who could walk, never helps. It adds a level of pressure that doesn't need to be there. It makes an already stressful situation worse. To say this comment to a nonambulatory child is worse. In addition to revealing the nurse as insensitive, it demonstrates that she didn't read Andreas's chart. Her speech provided me with information about her, and I knew that I didn't want her in the operating room. I was reassured when she left after accompanying us to the operating room.

I wrote about my experience with the hospital—both good and bad—on a questionnaire that the hospital sent after our experience. I wrote about our experience with the nurse. To the hospital's credit, a representative did call to ask me to identify the nurse. The representative told me that the example had already been used as a teaching tool for the nurses. I told her that if the situation had already been presented to the nurses, the nurse in question knew who she was, and I didn't need to identify her. The response of the hospital administrator was off target. What the hospital wished to do, it seemed to me, was to single out one nurse for reprimand. This was the logic that prevailed when the organization saw the behavior as coming from a rogue organizational member. I have tried to argue in this book that these behaviors are systematic issues within the medical culture. If we continue to see behaviors as aberrant, then change will never happen. I am arguing that this nurse's communication grows directly out of the medical culture. There will only be change when people within the medical culture see that their words are powerful and have a huge impact on the patients that they treat every day.

Some of what is routinely done within the medical culture is not only lacking in thought but also lacking in logic. After

Andreas seized and we visited a new neurologist, he suggested that Andreas have an EEG. He said that he needed to rule out that Andreas was having seizures of which I was unaware. I told him that I knew what Andreas's seizures looked like, and since he required our constant care, he was never alone. The night when he had the seizure, I jumped out of bed because I heard him making sounds that were not normal.

I agreed to go ahead and schedule the EEG. The doctor wrote on the prescription that Andreas should be sleep deprived prior to the test. I called the hospital to book the appointment. I asked if the receptionist could tell me what the doctor expected to see during the EEG. I was a little familiar with the EEG because Andreas had had so many while he was in the NICU.

She said, "I'm not going to go into specifics with you as to what we're looking for." She was clearly impatient with me and my questions.

I said, "Okay. Tell me why the doctor is asking for my son to be sleep deprived."

I didn't know exactly what to ask, but I was trying to understand. That question proved to be the correct one since it gave me the information that I needed.

"Because we will have a baseline reading, and when he falls asleep, we will be able to compare the two numbers," she explained.

Andreas would never fall asleep in the middle of the afternoon under any circumstances. He sometimes would awake at 2:00 a.m., and he would stay awake until bedtime that night. I could say with certainty that he was not going to fall asleep in a strange room with electrodes glued to his head. I always thought it unwise to wake a sleeping child, and it is especially unwise to wake a sleeping child who just had a seizure. Depriving Andreas of sleep didn't make sense to me, so I told the doctor that we weren't going to do it. He listened and accepted my response.

We arrived at the hospital at the designated time. We walked past the room where the EEGs were being performed on children. Mothers, looking like medical Madonnas cradling their infants in their arms, with babies hooked up to machines stared out as we made our way to the waiting room. We were directed to a small, cramped, dirty waiting room that had a television blaring. I went to use the restroom and had a sinking feeling in my stomach. When I returned, I told my husband that my inclination was to take Andreas and leave. I didn't want to put Andreas through an ordeal for the sake of performing a test. My instinct was that Andreas didn't need the EEG. If he did need it, I would have had the test done. My instinct, though, told me not to have any test performed at this hospital. The hospital appeared filthy, and the medical staff was curt. Looking at the other mothers and their children brought back many bad memories of Andreas's time in the neonatal unit. I wondered if he had any memories of that time too.

We never did have the EEG, and thankfully, Andreas never had another seizure. Since the birth of the twins, I tried to pay close attention to the messages that I received. If I enter a doctor's office, and I have a strong negative impression, I pay attention. I try not to dismiss it. I also watch Andreas, and if he is not at ease in the environment we're in, I pay attention. I no longer see the medical community as having something that I need, so I do not feel desperate. Recently, Andreas, my husband, and I visited a pediatrician who specializes in the use of hyperbaric oxygen therapy. The doctor sounded very promising to me because she has a daughter with cerebral palsy.

We were not impressed by our initial introduction to the medical staff and the office. Andreas immediately started to cry and look uncomfortable. Both my husband and I felt uncomfortable, although we did not say anything to each other. I felt very clearly that we should leave. I approached the front desk clerk and told her that we did not feel comfortable. Some weeks after this, I heard through the grapevine (it's a small community) that a little girl started to seize after receiving hyperbaric oxygen therapy from this doctor. Doctors usually schedule many sessions of the therapy and request prepayment. The girl seized after the first treatment, and the parents canceled subsequent appointments. Seizing is always a risk, but I heard that the doctor would not refund the parents for the canceled sessions.

This example demonstrates more a lack of ethics than a parting of thought and action seeming to defy common sense.

Andreas had acid reflux when he was a newborn. It became one of my full-time jobs to search out bottles and formula he could tolerate. I frequently had to change formulas because what he could tolerate always changed. After we weaned him from formula, we found that he did much better if he did not have dairy. We then found that he also does better if he doesn't have soy. The single recommendation that our doctors provided for babies with reflux is to give them an antacid. We did as the doctors suggested and placed Andreas on an antacid. It didn't help. Like many parents of children with cerebral palsy, we took Andreas to see a gastroenterologist. He suggested that we stay with the antacids and hope that Andreas outgrew the acid reflux. If it persisted, he told us, we could have a test performed during which a tube inserted down Andreas's throat would allow a closer look.

I didn't think that the options, as they were presented, were good enough. I took Andreas to see a naturopathic doctor who told me that antacids never work because they give the body the false message that there is not enough acid, and the body begins to make more. She told me to follow a supplement protocol that consisted of vitamins and probiotics (a product that introduces good bacteria into the system). Andreas started to improve.

The protocol worked for three years, and then the reflux started to flare up. I went back to the research. This has been my experience with Andreas. What his body needs always changes, so what works now will not necessarily work later.

In the midst of trying to remedy the reflux, and the constipation that usually goes along with it, I started to consult with a nutritionist. When the antacids were not working for Andreas, I did read the insert that comes with the product and learned that a side effect of taking the drug is constipation. The antacid that is frequently prescribed usually doesn't work, and it may worsen the condition. In addition, the use of an antacid may create or worsen constipation. Doctors seem to advocate antacids as the best cure for reflux, but I have never seen a child whose symptoms were relieved by the use of antacid.

I now know that Andreas's GI tract is a work in progress. Recently, I have begun to work with a new nutritionist, and the improvement in Andreas has been dramatic. His reflux has entirely gone away.

I don't expect the doctors to know everything. I do find it perplexing that when what the doctors offer doesn't work, I am left on my own to figure out what will improve my son's quality of life. I do find it troubling that doctors don't offer basic suggestions about responding naturally to a child's acid reflux and/or constipation issues.

In spite of the doctors' lack of helpfulness with regard to these conditions, most people that I encounter still ask, "What do the doctors say?"

Chapter 9
The Language of the Self-contained System or "The Locked Box"

Disconnected from Other Protocols

The previous chapter's theme—thought and action parting company—provides a good transition into a discussion of the language of the self-contained system. The medical culture does not seem to receive much feedback from other systems. It seems to do what it perceives to be correct, and the decisions about what is correct seem to be made within a vacuum. It has been frustrating to feel that I need to reinvent the wheel. I have talked with other mothers who have traveled the same rough road. For instance, I've never heard of a mother whose pediatrician told her to look into diet and the use of probiotics to manage reflux.

The gastroenterologist we consulted regarding Andreas's stomach problems demonstrated this resistance to ideas. I disclosed that, at the time, we'd removed gluten, soy, and dairy from Andreas's diet.

The doctor responded with sarcasm. He asked, "Is there anything left to feed him?"

This was asked as a rhetorical question. He wasn't waiting for me to answer him. He simply seemed to resist the fact that a change in a child's diet will affect his or her symptoms. This reaction seemed odd given the recent research produced within the medical field. In *The Second Brain*, Michael D. Gershon, MD, explores a new area of medicine called neurogastroenterology that recognizes a second brain in the bowel. "The seminal discovery," states Gershon, "that established its existence was the demonstration that the gut contains nerve cells that can 'go it alone'; that is, they can operate the organ without instructions from the brain or spinal cord" (Gershon 1998).

It's odd that research from within the field of medicine has pointed to connections between the brain and the gut, yet when I mentioned the connection during an office visit with a gastroenterologist, he resisted the knowledge. I am not the only parent commenting on this oddity. In *The Boy Who Loved Windows*, Stacey makes a similar observation.

She describes meeting with a gastroenterologist in this way:

> When Cliff [her husband] mentioned the idea that
> wheat and dairy might be detrimental to those with
> autism spectrum disorder, he [the doctor] grew visible
> angry. I mentioned a book I was reading …, which
> described the benefits of removing wheat and dairy for
> kids like Walker [her son]. He said, "There's no scientific
> proof to that notion at all. You give him anything you
> can. He's too small and frail for you to limit his diet"
> (Stacey 2004).

In *The Brain that Changes Itself*, Norman Doidge, MD, uses the idea of brain placidity to explore the resistance of the medical culture to let go of false ideas and embrace new theories.

He writes about how doctors perceived that once there was trauma to the brain, there was no turning back. He shows how researchers' experience with cases have proved otherwise. These early researchers could not get their work published. The medical culture held on to its beliefs, despite contrary evidence. (Doidge 2007) Doidge's work refashions the philosopher Schopenhauer's edict that new ideas on the landscape always follow the same trajectory. At first, people ignore the new idea, simply pretending it doesn't exist. Then, after they can no longer ignore the idea, they refute it. After people have refuted the idea, they treat it as common knowledge. People don't remember the history. They treat the claim as if it were a self-evident truth.

The idea that the brain is placid has now achieved the level of common knowledge within the medical community. Doctors now agree that the brain is highly plastic and can adapt, change, and grow after injury. There continues, however, to be a great divide between allopathic and homeopathic medicine. Doctors appear to insulate themselves from the homeopathic remedies that improve the quality of life for many children with disabilities.

I think that natural remedies may follow the same trajectory as all other ideas. For now, most medical doctors either ignore the helpful effects that come through homeopathic avenues or they refute the gains achieved through any other means but allopathic medicine. We may eventually come to a time where the beneficial effects from homeopathic means may be regarded as common knowledge. What I find interesting about these trajectories is the historical amnesia that comes with it.

Disconnected from the Self

To best exemplify the resistance of the medical culture to see itself, I'll share a story from another century. It is now well known that doctors initially refused to see that the lack of hand washing protocols before surgery was resulting in patients' deaths. In the early days of medical surgery, doctors would simply operate on a patient without washing his hands. When people suggested that the doctors may be causing deaths from this practice, doctors, for the most part, refused to believe it. I think that the medical culture, maybe more than other cultures, is more resistant to the idea that it may be doing more harm than good. I believe this attitude comes from training. Doctors are trained to help people, and that training is admirable. A side effect, however, can be the attitude that a doctor can do no wrong. I think that it's difficult for doctors within the existing medical culture to balance self-confidence and healthy self-questioning. If a doctor questions him or herself in an emergency situation, dire consequences may ensue. But not questioning how his or her decisions could be making a situation worse for a patient could result in a different set of consequences.

Chapter 10
The Language of Condescension
or "Professional Bullying"

Disconnected from Fellow Physicians

An article in the *New York Times*, entitled "In 'Sweetie' and 'Dear,' a Hurt beyond Insult for the Elderly" (Leland 2008), addresses the use of "elderspeak" within the medical culture. The article illustrates how medical professionals' tendency to address elderly people condescendingly has a negative consequence on the health of older people. There appears to be a dumbing down within the medical culture, and this is what the older people are reacting against. They resent, rightly so, doctors speaking to them disrespectfully.

Along with this dumbing down, the medical culture participates in "dumping down" when it comes to interns, who are routinely treated badly by their superiors. This seems to be a form of a rite of passage. Having passed through this ill treatment successfully, the newly minted physician can then pass on the poor treatment to the new incoming group of interns. And so it goes.

What the article doesn't say is that this bullying is part of medical culture. It seems to me that bullying is built in to the medical culture. A dumping down speech permeates the medical culture. The *Times* article suggests that the medical community's language is different from other settings because of the power we attribute to the words of the medical staff. Any time that bullying occurs, it is damaging, but bullying may be more so within the medical culture.

I don't think the article got it right. Bullying is not an aberration but, in fact, a part of the culture that is learned when an organizational member is initiated into the culture. There are people who do not bully within the medical culture, but I think these people resist this aspect of the culture. Most people, however, acquire the norms of their culture and recreate what they've been exposed to. Bullying within the medical culture does not necessarily happen because the people within the culture are mean-spirited. People within the medical culture bully others and speak down to others because doing so is part of their culture. They get away with this kind of talk because they have the weight of the culture behind them.

If we sincerely wish to reduce bullying within our larger culture, we need to first look at how our institutions systematically recreate bullying. I think that bullying is rampant in our culture, but we seem to isolate it to the playground. Children model what they see. Many children are exposed to bullying at home and/or in the classroom. They carry out that behavior toward other children.

Bullying is ego gratification and throwing around one's weight at the expense of someone else. There are several types of bullies. Some bullies use brute physical threat or force like that seen on the playground. Some teachers and doctors are intellectual bullies and attempt to shame their students for not knowing or asking questions. Last, there are the emotional bullies who use other people's vulnerabilities to further weaken them.

It takes a strong person to ward off bullying. Sometimes, the unconscious parent can even bully his or her own child. It takes vigilance to resist feeling superior to those who are most vulnerable. Doctors need to be very vigilant about bullying because bullying is built into their culture, and daily they may treat those who are physically, emotionally, and intellectually vulnerable.

The cultural counterbalance for bullying is empathy. If one can truly place him or herself in the position of others, there would not be bullying. If teachers could remember their own struggles as students, they would be less inclined to use intellectual bullying as a tactic. If doctors could imagine how they would feel being at the mercy of people or practices beyond their control, they would not bully their patients.

Chapter 11
The Language of Generalization
or "Kids Like These ..."

Disconnected from the Patient

Andreas's GI tract has been an issue for us since he was an infant. Over the Christmas holiday in 2008, Andreas's stomach problems worsened. We've always been able to relieve his reoccurring problem with gas by massage and the use of a hot water bottle. The weekend after Christmas, the situation became worse. Andreas had gas, constipation, and, on top of everything else, he picked up a stomach virus. He was waking up every hour crying in pain. At 3:00 a.m., my husband took Andreas to the emergency room where they x-rayed his stomach and told us nothing else appeared wrong other than that he was constipated. The doctor instructed us to give Andreas a child enema and infant mylocon.

We had only given Andreas an enema once before and mylocon hadn't worked when Andreas had colic as a baby, but I was willing to try it again. The next day, we gave Andreas the enema and the mylocon. He experienced some relief, but only partially. At the end of the following day, I spoke to Andreas's pediatrician and told her Andreas was still in discomfort.

"And that's after you have been giving him adult stool softener and adult suppositories?" she replied.

I explained that I wasn't giving him adult products and that no one had ever mentioned that before. At that point, I would have given him anything to make him more comfortable. After following the pediatrician's suggestion, Andreas was the most comfortable he had been in a week.

The day Andreas contracted the stomach virus, I was going to meet with a new nutritionist. I canceled the appointment because Andreas was not well. Prior to this current crisis, we'd stopped Andreas's probiotic because his pediatrician said that they can cause gas. Up until then, the probiotics were doing a beautiful job managing the gas. Prior to this episode, we'd also started Andreas on a new digestive enzyme and placed him back on aloe juice. We were also following a gluten-free diet.

Once Andreas was more comfortable, I talked with the new nutritionist, who provided lots of good suggestions, and we booked an appointment with the head of pediatric gastroenterology. We'd seen Dr. Bernard when Andreas was six months old, and he had told us that Andreas would outgrow his acid reflux. He'd given us no alternative treatment options to antacid mediation.

I'd taken Andreas off the antacid mediation when he was an infant after I noticed it was not helping him and after I read on the insert that the medication causes constipation. A holistic doctor I consulted at the time told me that taking antacids gives the body the message to make more acid.

I made the appointment with Dr. Bernard hoping he'd be of more use this time. He wasn't. I'd been responding to Andreas's condition for six years and each protocol we'd introduced had brought with it some improvement. I discovered a condition called gastro paresis that can be caused by acid reflux (and the use of antacid medication, among other causes), and the symptoms fit Andreas. I'd wanted to speak to Dr. Bernard about the possibility of gastro paresis applying to Andreas. Once again, I felt that if I had a label that applied to Andreas, I could make changes for that condition.

When I asked Dr. Bernard about gastro paresis, he said that the diagnostic procedures were invasive (they are) and noted that, even if Andreas had gastro paresis, there was nothing we could do about it. This wasn't the first time I'd heard that from a physician, and I knew it couldn't be true. From the little bit of research I'd begun, I'd learned about changes I could make if Andreas had this condition. Dr. Bernard said that, in all likelihood, Andreas did have gastro paresis, but he neither educated us more about it nor recommended anything we could do about it.

Dr. Bernard examined Andreas and told us to meet him in his office. The examination consisted of him feeling Andrea's abdomen and doing a rectal exam to see if his bowels were empty. We told him that we were unsure if Andreas was gaining weight since three scales (one in the pediatrician's office, one in the hospital the night before, and one in this doctor's office) showed different results. Dr. Bernard never bothered to double-check Andreas's weight during the visit. He also never bothered to introduce the person shadowing him, whom I assume was an intern. What I most remember of her is that she looked petrified. She was without affect and said nothing other than "he will be with you in a minute."

When we arrived in Dr. Bernard's office, we found him seated at his desk writing prescriptions and looking at the computer screen. The intern was seated against the wall. He was writing prescription after prescription without saying a word to us. I looked at the intern, and that's when she spoke: "He will be with you in a minute."

I finally said, "I hope those prescriptions aren't for Andreas."

"No," the doctor said, "this is for something [I don't think he used the word *patient*] else that I have to take care of."

Later, Dr. Bernard told us the same thing he'd said in the examination room about how constipation occurs. At this point Andreas started to cry and my husband left the room with him.

"Are we done here?" I asked.

"I haven't given you my protocol I recommend," Dr. Bernard replied. He showed me a generic piece of paper that I assume he gives to everyone. The paper instructed me that frosted mini-wheats contain five to six grams of fiber. I took the piece of paper without saying thank you because I felt that he'd given me nothing meaningful.

When I didn't say thank you, he said, "Bye now."

I left the office less angry than I'd left other doctor offices in the past because I had gotten used to this practice. Dr. Bernard was not helpful. On the drive home, I asked my husband if he thought I was expecting too much to have wanted Dr. Bernard to tell us that the prescriptions he was writing weren't for us instead of letting us just sit there. We had told him in the examining room that we'd been dealing with Andreas's GI problems for six years, the current flair-up for a week, and the death of my husband's mother the day before (when he asked if our parents were living). Was it expecting too much to think that this well-educated man should know better? I wondered about what the intern was learning about how to treat her patients?

My husband and I come away from these appointments with different views of reality. He says that I am expecting too much, and I say that he accepts too little. I commented to my husband that I felt this doctor had categorized me negatively because I told him that I removed many elements from my son's diet and that I'd done my own research. My husband thinks that I tell the medical professionals we meet with too much information. According to him, the interaction between doctor and patient is a dance where you let them tell you information without disclosing any. I don't see medicine as a dance. I'm trying to help my son, and I think the best way to do that is by full disclosure.

My husband thinks that I gave Dr. Bernard too much information, and the information that I gave him made it easy for him to draw certain assumptions about me.

My husband thought that I gave the doctor cause for seeing me as "a New Age mother who thinks that making dietary changes will help her son." He believes that during a doctor visit you should answer only the questions asked without volunteering further information. He thinks this is the best way to avoid doctors forming a stereotype about the parent and then having this stereotype getting in the way of rendering a diagnosis.

I understand my husband's point of view. It is not, however, my way.

I told Dr. Bernard about Andreas's diet because I wanted him to know the truth.

Unfortunately, Dr. Bernard saw "just another kid with cerebral palsy" instead of seeing Andreas. He said several times during the visit "What you see in kids like these is …"

I don't want to hear about "kids like these." I want to hear what you can tell me about Andreas.

To return to the theme of this book, the question I heard many times during Andreas's latest crisis was "What does the doctor say?"

Aside from the good advice from Andreas's pediatrician about evacuation, Dr. Bernard said very little.

I received several pages of suggestions from the nutritionist, but no one asks, "What does the nutritionist say?" The insurance company will reimburse us for 80 percent of the three hundred dollars we spent on Dr. Bernard and will pay nothing on the expense for the nutritionist.

After our visit with Dr. Bernard, I consulted *Smart Medicine for a Healthier Child*. The authors write about the contraindications of mineral oil (the gastroenterologist's recommendation). They note that prolonged use of mineral oil can cause inflammation of the liver, spleen, and abdominal lymph nodes. Mineral oil can interfere with the body's absorption of vitamins A and D. Also the lubricant can be dangerous if it accidentally goes down the windpipe and enters the lungs (Zand, Walton, and Rountree 1994). This last point is especially important to note when treating a child with cerebral palsy since swallowing may be a problem.

Dr. Bernard never asked if Andreas had swallowing difficulties.

I followed up on all the recommendations offered by the nutritionist, and Andreas is doing much better. I left the meeting with Dr. Bernard mystified as to why a GI specialist wasn't more help in curing my son's constipation. In part, I think his inability to help was a result of his assumption that constipation goes along with cerebral palsy and there is nothing that can be done about it. Other doctors have since suggested that this is not the specialty of a GI doctor. My question is, then, if constipation is not in a GI specialist's area of expertise, why do pediatricians refer patients suffering from constipation to the GI specialist?

As to Dr. Bernard in particular, other doctors have noted that he's fine to work with if your child is suffering from Crohn's disease. My question is this: How does a parent sort through this labyrinth of caveats?

I also reflected on the disconnection of this doctor. He seemed to me to be lacking a connection with his intern, with my husband and me, with my child, and with the alternative health literature on ways to relieve constipation. As I see it, no one gained from this office visit.

Chapter 12
The Language of Passive
Aggression or "I Really Do Not
Want to Treat This Child"

Disconnected from the Impact of One's Words within the Therapeutic Setting

At times, the medical culture spills over to the therapeutic setting. The situation with Andreas's speech pathologist had been building for several weeks. I chose to overlook the last-minute cancellations, the dirty office, and the odd interpersonal encounters with the therapist. I overlooked them because Andreas was happy with Alexandra. I drove him to Connecticut twice a week where Andreas met with Alexandra, or her assistants, for two-hour sessions. I chose to overlook the difficulties with Alexandra because Andreas always came out of the sessions happy and alert. The relationship mutually dissolved one Thursday afternoon.

I arrived on time for our one o'clock appointment. Alexandra was late. I saw her car pass so I figured that she was parking her car in the back parking lot. As she walked through the hall, she stopped to chat with her colleague. When Alexandra arrived in the waiting room, she offered no apology for being late. I chose to say nothing about her lateness. I told her that the school district and I wanted to videotape Andreas in his therapy sessions because we wanted to use this video as part of an end-of-the-school-year awards ceremony. Alexandra told me that she did not like to be videotaped. I explained that I could just film Andreas so she need not worry.

As I pushed Andreas into the treatment room, Alexandra said, "I'm thinking about the videotaping and whether or not I like it. I like to think about things. That's the way I am."

Previous to this, Alexandra had displayed what I would call a power play, and I chalked it up to interpersonal awkwardness. Alexandra had canceled one morning, and I received the call at 10:00 a.m. Andreas had already left for his day of therapy. He was to have his session with Laurie (his education therapist) and then Laurie would feed him lunch. I had an appointment that afternoon, so my husband agreed to pick up Andreas from Laurie and take him to Alexandra. A cancellation at 10:00 a.m. changed the entire day. When I arrived for the next session, I wanted to tell Alexandra that I would prefer to know about cancellations at 9:00 a.m. instead of 10:00 a.m.

"I'm going to say one thing about the cancellation, and then I'll be done," I began.

"After you speak, I'll have my say, and then we'll be done!" she responded.

I was dumbfounded by this response because it sounded so juvenile.

Her last say was, "I hear you. Now we're done."

I left the office to sit in my car in front of the office as I usually did on Tuesdays and Thursdays. I called my husband to tell him that I thought that the relationship with Alexandra was ending. At that point, I was getting fed up with Alexandra. I knew of another mother who had stopped bringing her son to Alexandra because she grew tired of the no-shows at school and the last-minute cancellations. Alexandra had also failed to show up for meetings with Andreas's therapists. Part of her job, as contracted by the school district, was to make sure that the technology—in other words, Andreas's communication device—was integrated into all aspects of his therapy. The school district paid Andreas's therapists directly. One negative experience that Alexandra and I had was about money.

I was on my way to Alexandra's, and her secretary called to say that Alexandra was canceling because the school district hadn't paid her for a while. I called the administrator, and everything was resolved in time for Andreas to make his appointment. Looking back, I should have ended our relationship with Alexandra then. Alexandra's actions told me a lot of information about her, but I forged ahead because I perceived that she had something that we needed. I also forged ahead because Alexandra was a vast improvement on the previous augmentative speech therapist that we'd had.

I spoke with Andreas's other therapist and discovered that none of them had been paid during this period. The other therapists took the situation in stride and understood that it had to do with the school district's billing cycle. They said that they knew the cycle would catch up, and they knew to build in for this lapse when working with school districts. They were all appalled that Alexandra would take out her frustration with the school on Andreas.

When I arrived at the appointment, I told Alexandra, "I'm going to tell you something from the viewpoint of the mother. How you handled the situation concerning the bills was poor. It was not good that you didn't tell me what was going on and then had you secretary call me to cancel."

Alexandra said, "I had to do something."

"But what you chose to do wasn't good," I replied.

Her last words were, "I hear you."

When I reflected upon this experience with Alexandra, I realized that there were warning signs I choose not to heed. I chose to stay, even though I tell myself I should leave bad situations as soon as I realize they're not working out; I know from previous experience that the question is never "why did I leave?" but instead "why didn't I get out sooner?"

I believe that Alexandra really didn't want to spend her time treating patients. Much of the energy and work of Alexandra and her office staff were spent on preparing for a big upcoming conference on autism. I think that Alexandra would have much preferred to spend her time working the lecture circuit. In fact, she did reveal as much one afternoon. She said that she envisioned spending her time going from one speaking engagement to the next.

I am detailing what happened leading up to and during our last session with Alexandra because I think it's instructive in understanding what can happen when a practitioner's heart is not in her work. In other words, my experience with Alexandra spoke to her intention. I do not think that Alexandra wanted to work with Andreas, and I chose not to pay attention to the warning signs that appeared along the way. Intention is a tricky communication concept because the listener sometimes needs to go beyond the words to listen for the intention.

Sometimes, the speaker doesn't intend to hurt the other with his or her words, and it's important to hear that intention. Here, Alexandra intended on getting out of treating Andreas and the school contract she'd signed. I think that she thought that the only way to do this was to blame Andreas and me. This is exactly what she did.

On the afternoon on which our relationship finally came to an end, I checked in on Andreas midway into the session. I always checked in on him since Alexandra and her staff didn't look after Andreas the way his other therapists did. On occasion, I would check in on him, and Andreas would have had a bowel movement and the person working with him hadn't thought to come get me. I would come into the treatment room midway so that I could change him, give him something to drink, and let him stretch out a bit.

This day, I was giving Andreas a drink as Alexandra began to explain herself. "The last couple of weeks have been difficult," she told me. "Andreas has been spitting up a lot. I need to worry if I have paper towels and make sure that everything remains clean."

During this time, I remained quiet, holding Andreas's cup as he sipped from a straw.

Alexandra continued, "Now, you want to videotape, and I'm already dealing with all of these interruptions in the session.

I'm not comfortable with body fluids. Body fluids are not my thing."

I could feel my anger welling up, but at this time, I kept my anger under control. "Alexandra," I said, "I don't think that bodily fluids are anyone's thing, but I'm not going to speak to you about this now. I'm going to finish giving Andreas his drink, and then I'm taking him home."

As she walked me to the door, she asked if I was taking his communication device with me. I said that I was. I felt that this question was a covert way of asking if we were ever coming back. I say this because Andreas had a week off from school the upcoming week, and we'd discussed Alexandra keeping the device over the school break. By the time I left her office, my hands were shaking with anger. I knew that I was not going back to Alexandra, but I was concerned because I knew that augmentative communication therapists were hard to find. One of Andreas's other therapists had suggested that I hold on to Alexandra until I could find a replacement. I knew that this was a poor practice for any relationship. When it's time to end the relationship, it's time.

On the way home from Alexandra's, I called my friend Lisa. Lisa had referred me to Alexandra, and I knew that she'd severed her own relationship with Alexandra some months prior because, as she put it, she could no longer take Alexandra's unprofessional behavior. Lisa told me that she thought she had finally found a replacement therapist after several months of looking.

When I arrived home, I called the chair of our school district's committee for special education (CSE). The chairperson had known of Alexandra's cancellations, but she hadn't heard about any of Alexandra's other unprofessional behaviors. She was surprised that I wanted to stop working with Alexandra. The chairperson, who was and is extremely supportive, said, "We have a contract with Alexandra until the end of the year."

I hadn't thought about the school district being contractually obligated to keep Alexandra or pay her until the end of the school year. When I hung up the phone, I thought about ways that I could show that Alexandra, on several occasions, violated the contract by being late, canceling, having assistants work with Andreas without our permission (or even a proper introduction), and giving away his time slot when another school district needed to schedule a meeting during his regular time. I even thought about reviewing the records to see if Alexandra had submitted for payment during any time when she'd canceled since the contract stipulated that payment be for services rendered only.

I never had to pursue any of these loopholes because Alexandra soon called the CSE chairperson. She recast what had happened to suit her intention. She wanted out, but it seemed that she could not just come out and say it. According to Alexandra, "Andreas has been sick for the last couple of sessions. He had been vomiting during our sessions. I told the mother that I'm not comfortable with bodily fluids. I'm not a doctor, and I'm not set up to deal with this. The mother's response is to give him some water."

The CSE chairperson asked Alexandra if she wished to terminate the contract, and she said she did.

Alexandra, in order to get out the contract, chose her words carefully. Words create worlds, and in this case, Alexandra changed "spitting up" to "vomiting." She suggested that Andreas was sick, and I was ignoring the issue.

She painted me as a neglectful mother. Her word choice implied that I was the type of mother who would send a sick child to therapy. Andreas was not sick, and if he was, I would never have sent him to therapy. He was experiencing reflux. It had previously been under control with the use of supplements, and it had flared up again. Alexandra knew that I was struggling to resolve this and had put all of my energy into resolving his stomach issues. I had disclosed all of this to her, so I perceived her reaction as particularly heartless.

More importantly, I hated that she spoke the way she did in front of Andreas. Throughout our therapy sessions, Alexandra had told me that she thought Andreas understood everything. Now I wondered, *Did she think he understood everything and spoke these words in front of him anyway?*

She told me during our last session that she thought I could appreciate honesty and that she could not live without being honest. This is a strategy that people who display passive aggression employ. They use words that cut to the bone and then say, "I was only being honest."

In this situation, I didn't appreciate a therapist telling me, in front of Andreas, that something he was doing, which he had no control over, disgusted her. Sometimes, people continually give children who have disabilities messages that what they're doing isn't okay. In this case, Alexandra—someone who was supposedly there on Andreas's behalf—gave him the message that something he was doing that he wasn't in control of was disgusting. Therapists like Alexandra are toxic to children with disabilities because what these kids least need is to receive messages that they are inadequate from people who are supposed to serve them.

As I noted, I was reluctant to end therapy sessions with Alexandra because she had been a vast improvement from our previous augmentative communication therapist, Natalie. Natalie, too, would cancel on us, not notifying us of the cancellation until we'd showed up for the session. Her office was also dirty, but in addition, it was cramped, and maneuvering Andreas's wheelchair wasn't easy. In contrast to Alexandra, Natalie could never engage Andreas. He looked miserable during these sessions and would often look at me as if to say, "Get me out of here."

I didn't listen to him for too long. Natalie showed him the same mind-numbing video during each session. She would sip her coffee and call Andreas by the wrong name. Once, she told him that a fire truck was an ambulance. She wasn't present with him, and he seemed to know it.

Because of Natalie, I was pleased when we found Alexandra. At least, I rationalized, Andreas is happy and engaged with Alexandra. She never called him by a wrong name, but she would consistently misspell his name on reports and on his communication device. When I called this error to her attention, she acted as if it was the first time she'd heard of her mistake. I knew that she was being disingenuous since it drove his other therapists crazy and they had called it to her attention.

The use of passive aggressive language is a tip-off that there's a problem. People who use the language of passive aggression are usually angry. I don't know if Alexandra was angry; I do think that she was spending her time doing something she really didn't want to do. Ultimately, Andreas wasn't going to be served by someone who wanted to be doing something else. He needed professionals who were committed to their work and to him.

Thankfully, Andreas has a group of therapists who are not only professionally gifted but who give their hearts to their work.

The conclusion of this story with Alexandra has a happy ending. I now say that the termination of our relationship with Alexandra was one of the best things that ever happened to us. Andreas had the following week off from school. By the next week, we had a new therapist. Marcie, the therapist Lisa referred me to, turned out to be more technically savvy than Alexandra, connected with Andreas better that Alexandra had, and came to our house twice a week for his sessions.

As of the writing of this book, Andreas is still seeing Marcie. Andreas has a little bit more breathing room in his schedule since we're not commuting to Connecticut twice a week. Marcie is teaching him how to use a communication device, she's responsive to the school district in terms of reports and other issues, and she's working to bring us all up to speed concerning the available technology that is available. On top of all this, she and Andreas laugh their way through the two-hour therapy sessions.

Conclusion

In this book, I have written about how we construct worlds through words. We all have the opportunity to choose our words, but frequently we do not. We sometimes are overtaken by our own inertia, and we run on scripts we have not written. When I do choose my words, however, the way I choose to talk about something or someone creates a world for both my listener and me. This is why I need to pay close attention to the words I use because, through them, I am choosing where I live.

One of the most powerful examples of someone finding the strength to construct his own reality with words is found in *Man's Search for Meaning* by Viktor Frankl. Frankl was a psychiatrist who developed his psychological theory of logotherapy from his time in a Nazi concentration camp. He speaks about how a man in the camp stole a piece of bread. The authorities found out about the incident and asked that the guilty man be given up. Frankl states, "Naturally, the two thousand five hundred men preferred to fast" (Frankl 1985). The condition Frankl is describing is the scarcity of food. The language he uses to describe this condition has powerful ramifications. If he had chosen the word *starve* to describe the condition, he would have implied that the men were victims. If the men had seen themselves as victims, they wouldn't have seen their ability to make choices. But even in describing this unbearable situation, Frankl uses language to show that the men had the power to unite and act in accordance with a higher principle. The shift from the word *starve* to the word *fast* is a shift from victimization to autonomy.

The most important element in Frankl's statement is the element of choice. We all choose the words we use, and the words create worlds. Cultures are no different. Cultures are created by words. In this book, I have provided an analysis of the words doctors use to examine what kind of culture is created. Rather than seeing the consumers of health care as its victims, I see us as co-creators of the medical culture. We all play a role in the recreation of medical culture. One way we contribute to the medical culture as it exists now is by asking the question: What do the doctors say? Asking this question reinforces the existing hierarchy where the doctor, who knows, is on top. This question is so commonplace that we do not pay attention to the function it provides. One way to show how this question affects us is to juxtapose it with alternative questions. What if, for instance, we asked, "What have you and your doctor explored as potential remedies to your condition?" This one small shift would place the patient, or the patient's parents, into the health care equation.

The list of language patterns, while not exhaustive, may serve as a starting place to decipher aspects of the medical culture. The list is meant to provide patients or parents with ways to identify and speak about medical culture. Talking about a culture as a whole can be difficult because, when you think of a culture, you often think of it in terms of general impressions. It's helpful to break the culture down into the individual pieces that combine to give you those impressions. To this end, I have provided the following list of features that cumulatively create medical culture:

- I-focused talk

- Metaphors that objectify the patient

- Use of different labels to justify one's intention

- Removing the patient or parent from the communication transaction

- Constructing the person acting as the health care advocate as an obstacle

- The use of ambiguity

- The use of thoughtless language

- The quality of being impervious to criticism from outside the culture

- The use of condescending talk

- The use of generalizations

- The style of passive aggression

I know that my analysis of the medical culture is not complimentary. I'm not critiquing medicine but, instead, focusing on medical culture. I think that the medical culture that all of us help to create is toxic and does not serve any of us—or I should say most of us.

The current culture does seem to serve the insurance companies and the pharmaceutical industry.

I consulted a malpractice attorney because I believe that the hospital harmed Andreas by giving him prophylactic antibiotics while he was in the NICU. The lawyer explained that the use of antibiotics in this case was usual protocol. He said that I would have a better chance of establishing a legal case if the doctors had not administered antibiotics.

The medical literature I consulted advised physicians to wait and see before treating a newborn with prophylactic antibiotics (Taeusch, Ballard, and Gleason 2004). Andreas was not manifesting any symptoms when he was given the drugs, but the doctors gave them to him because they'd given the drugs to his brother. They could have easily waited and watched Andreas closely; he was already in the NICU to be near his brother. I am sure that fear of a lawsuit was one of the chief operating factors that influenced the doctors to give Andreas drugs in the first place. It is not comforting to imagine that health care professionals made a decision concerning my son's health based on economics. If this is true, the decision had nothing to do with a concern for his well-being.

As a consumer of health care, I find the current medical culture to be disconnected—from the patient, from areas of specialization and medicine, and from complementary forms of health care. In the introduction, I stated that medical culture would be greatly improved by a rhetoric of connection. A rhetoric of connection is established when doctor and patient discover ways to connect in the collaborative work of healing. The current system, as practiced in many medical offices that I visited, does not produce good care. I visited too many doctors who never looked at my son during an examination and either looked at a computer screen or his or her notes. It seems to me that a medical culture of disconnection produces doctors who fail to look, listen, and touch. These are doctors who are cut off from their own senses. It's no wonder their diagnoses and prognoses are nonsense. There are, of course, doctors who are very sensitive to the information that their senses provide, but my argument is that these doctors go against the medical culture in which they've been trained. These are doctors who subvert the culture in which they perform in order to do good work. These are the exceptional doctors.

I know that several medical schools are attempting to remedy the existing medical culture by providing courses in communication to their medical students. Some medical schools offer classes on listening, empathy, and medical narratives or storytelling. There are, I think, two issues with these offerings. One, communication education is an easy thing to do poorly. Merely placing a communication course within a program isn't enough. Doctors need to learn that much of what they do is communication-oriented, and the responsibility that goes along with being a communicator, especially within medicine, is great. Two, I think that medical schools need to address how communication creates a medical culture. Merely teaching communication skills is not going to create change.

One of the best examples I can offer of what a rhetoric of connection looks like is provided through film. *The Diving Bell and the Butterfly* is a film adaptation from Jean-Dominique Bauby's book depicting his story. Bauby was the editor in chief of the French *Elle* magazine when he suffered a stroke that left him with locked-in syndrome. Locked-in syndrome is when the person's cognitive function remains intact, but he or she is unable to speak or move. The person is literally trapped inside of an uncooperative body. With extreme patience and perseverance, Bauby and his speech pathologist realized that he could communicate by blinking one eye. The speech pathologist would recite the alphabet, and Bauby would blink on the desired letter.

He dictated an entire book that way—letter by letter. Bauby's story, as shown through Julian Schnabel's film, illustrates what can happen when health care professionals are motivated by their will to do whatever it takes to establish connection (Bauby 1998).

Reference List

Bauby, Jean-Dominique. 1998. *The Diving Bell and the Butterfly*. Jeremy Leggart, trans. New York: Vintage Books.

Beck, Martha. 2000. *Expecting Adam*. New York: Berkley Books, 220.

Doidge, Norman. 2007. *The Brain that Changes Itself*. New York: Viking.

Edelson, Miriam. 2000. *My Journey with Jake: A Memoir of Parenting and Disability*. Toronto, Canada: Between the Lines, 64.

Gershon, Michael D. 1998. *The Second Brain*. New York: Harper Collins, 3.

Gordon, Serena. Newborns in intensive care often exposed to pain. *US News and World Report*, 1 July 2008.

Frankl, Viktor E. 1985 *Man's Search for Meaning*. New York: Pocket Books, 102.

Leland, John. 2008. In "sweetie" and "dear," a hurt beyond insult for the elderly, *The New York Times*, 7 October 2008:1 and A18.

Leonhart, David. 2009. Dr. James will make it better. *The New York Times Magazine*, 8 November 2009: 32–47.

Parikh, Rahul K. 2008. Showing the patient the door, permanently. *The New York Times*, 10 June 2008: F6.

Rosenthal, Robert and Lenore Jacobson. *Pygmalion in the Classroom*. New York: Irvington, 1992, expanded edition.

Stacey, Patricia. 2004. *The Boy Who Loved Windows*. Cambridge, MA: Da Capo Press, 206.

Saul, Stephanie. 2009. The gift of life, and its price: Fertility treatments bring more twins and premature births. *The New York Times*, October 11, 2009: 1, 26–27.

Taeusch, William H., Roberta A. Ballard, and Christina A. Gleason. 2004. *Avery's Diseases of the Newborn*, 8th ed. Amsterdam: Elsevier, 328.

Zand, Janet, Rachel Walton, and Bob Rountree 1994. *Smart Medicine for a Healthier Child*. Garden City, NY: Avery Publishing Group.